JUICING FOR BEGINNERS

The Full Beginners' Approach To Weight
Loss, Health, And Wellness.

By

Mary Langley

TABLE OF CONTENTS

<u>Liver Cleansing Tonic</u>
<u>Blast Of Beet Berry</u>
<u>Juice of cucumber</u>

Introduction

Hello and welcome to the juicing world! Fruits and vegetables can be consumed in liquid form by juicing, which is a common and healthy practice. It entails squeezing the juice out of fresh vegetables while discarding the pulp and fiber. This method delivers a concentrated dose of nutrients easily and enjoyably, enabling you to absorb important vitamins, minerals, and antioxidants more effectively.

If you're new to juicing, this guide will assist you in beginning your juicing adventure by offering crucial advice and details to maximize your juicing experience.

Health Advantages: Juicing has several health advantages, including better digestion, a strengthened immune system, more energy, and radiant skin. Fresh juices' rich nutrient content can help assist in healthy weight management and general well-being.

Selecting a Juicer: Different varieties of juicers, including centrifugal, masticating, and cold press juicers, are available. Each has benefits and price ranges. A centrifugal juicer is a fantastic option for beginners because it is reasonably priced and simple to operate.

When choosing produce, go for a mix of vibrant fruits and vegetables to make juices that are well-balanced and nutrient-rich. Include foods like berries, apples, cucumbers, spinach, kale, oranges, spinach, and beets. If organic produce is not available, properly wash and clean your fruits and veggies before juicing. Organic produce is preferred.

Produce Preparation: To eliminate any dirt or residue, rinse your fruits and vegetables in cool water. Before juicing, you might need to peel some fruits like oranges and pineapples. To enhance juice extraction from leafy greens, bundle them tightly or fold them together before feeding them into the juicer.

Juicing techniques: Start with softer produce, such as leafy greens, then work your way up to tougher fruits and vegetables. This ensures the best juice output and prevents blockage. To maintain a smooth juicing process, avoid filling the feed funnel of the juicer.

Finding the right flavor balance for you means experimenting with various fruit and vegetable pairings. For added flavor and health advantages, juice a little lemon or add a tiny piece of ginger.

Consuming Juice: To maintain the most nutritious content, freshly produced juice should be drank right away. If you must preserve it, do so for up to 24 hours in the refrigerator in an airtight container. Juices should be shaken well before consumption because they could separate over time.

Be mindful that juices lack the fiber found in entire fruits and vegetables, although juicing can be highly nutritious. As a result, rather than replacing a healthy diet, they ought to supplement it. In addition, fruit-heavy juices should only be consumed in moderation due to their concentrated sugar content, especially if you have concerns about your blood sugar levels.

Take Note of Your Body: Pay attention to how juicing affects your body. Fresh juices may initially cause stomach disturbances in some people, but this is typical as your body gets used to the new nutrients.

Juicing can be a useful supplement to a healthy diet and lifestyle, but it is important to keep in mind that it is not a miraculous cure for all health problems. To find your favorite juices, have fun experimenting with different recipes and blends. Congratulations on becoming healthier and more energetic with the help of juicing!

Chapter 1: The Basics

Fresh fruit Juice or vegetable juice is ground, squeezed, or pressed to extract their juice during the juicing process. It's a term used now to describe a centuries-old practice of pressing picked fruits to swiftly access their nutrients.

Juices can be a useful beverage to add more nutrients to your diet and encourage weight loss.

However, Certain liquids are low in fiber and high in sugar, which can increase your calorie consumption and eventually result in weight gain.

This essentially applies to a wide variety of juices purchased from stores, which are frequently loaded with sugar, artificial flavors, and preservatives.

Fortunately, you can produce a variety of tasty and healthful juices at home with just a few basic ingredients and a juicer.

Alternatively, a blender is an option. This approach is preferable since it keeps more fiber, which can help you feel fuller and control your hunger.

Advantages of juicing

Due to their liquid form and increased concentration levels, juicing fruits and vegetables can aid your body in more effectively absorbing their maximal nutritional value. Fresh fruit and vegetable juice can offer a variety of necessary vitamins and minerals for the healthy operation of your body's systems.

For good cause, juicing has been dubbed one of the year's healthiest trends. Juicing has various health advantages that can improve your overall well-being and energy levels. It's also a simple method to obtain your daily dosage of vitamins minerals and fibers that are essential for good health.

Many different types of juices are available on the market, including freshly pressed homemade juices and pre-made juices found in stores. Freshly pressed homemade juices can be made from fruits and vegetables like apples, pineapples, beets, kale, and spinach, depending on the ingredients you have on hand. Pre-made juices usually contain a combination of fruits, vegetables, and nuts, ranging from sweet fruit juices to earthy green juices.

One benefit of juicing is that it's a convenient and delicious way to add superfoods like ginger, turmeric, and garlic into your diet. Superfoods can provide additional benefits like aiding digestion and boosting immunity, which is important for your overall health.

Drinking juice increases your daily intake of dietary fiber, helping to promote healthy digestion and even reducing the risk of heart disease. Fiber keeps you healthy, which can help with weight loss goals.

Drinking freshly prepared juice encourages gastrointestinal regularity. Juice consumption uses less energy from your body for digestion because there is no chewing involved, which may lead to fewer digestive problems. Freshly squeezed juices regularly consumed can also assist in supplying vital vitamins and minerals to help avoid diseases like diabetes and high blood pressure.

Chapter 2 Fruits And Their Health Benefits.

Fruits are a great source of fiber as well as important vitamins and minerals. Antioxidants and flavonoids are included in various types of fruits, which are good for your health.

A diet rich in fruits and vegetables can lower a person's risk of diabetes, cancer, inflammation, heart disease, and other diseases.

The body receives nutrients and antioxidants by consuming a variety of fruits, which can improve general health and lower the risk of disease. There are many other options, but oranges, blueberries, apples, avocados, and bananas are among the best.

Apple
Apples, one of the most popular fruits, are packed with nutrients.

They contain a lot of soluble and insoluble fiber, including cellulose, hemicellulose, and pectin. These facilitate healthy digestion, support gut and heart health, and help you control your blood sugar levels.
Additionally, they are a strong source of vitamin C and plant polyphenols, which are disease-preventive substances found in plants. Regular apple consumption may reduce your

chances of neurological problems, cancer, heart disease, stroke, and being overweight.

You should eat the apple to get the most advantages because the majority of the polyphenols are found just below the skin.

Blueberries: The antioxidant and anti-inflammatory effects of blueberries are widely known.

They are high in anthocyanin, a flavonoid and plant pigment that gives blueberries their distinctive blue-purple color. This substance aids in the battle against disease-causing, cell-damaging free radicals.
A diet high in anthocyanins has been linked to several health advantages, including a reduced risk of type 2 diabetes, heart disease, obesity, high blood pressure, certain types of cancer, and cognitive decline.

For instance, a study with over 200,000 participants found that for every 17 grams of berries high in anthocyanins taken daily, there was a 5% reduction in the incidence of type 2 diabetes.

Elderberries, bilberry, blackberry chokeberries, and cherries are other berries strong in anthocyanins.

Fruit is healthy, but which fruit is the healthiest? Include as many different types of fruit as you can because they are all healthy.

"A daily apple keeps the doctor away," as the adage goes.

Healthcare professionals are aware that fruit is a delightful, incredibly nutrient-dense, and practical supplement to any diet. You might be uncertain about which fruit to choose because there are more than 2,000 types available.

Each type of fruit gives a special combination of nutrients and health advantages. The secret is to consume fruits of varied colors, as each color offers a unique collection of beneficial elements.

Here are the top 20 fruit choices that are the healthiest to consume often.

Bananas

Bananas have advantages beyond their potassium concentration. Bananas contain 7% of the Daily Value (DV) of potassium in addition to other nutrients.

27% of the DV for vitamin B6
12% of the DV for vitamin C
8% of the DV for magnesium
Additionally, they give a variety of phytosterols and polyphenols, two plant chemicals that are good for your general health. Additionally, they contain a lot of prebiotics, a type of fiber that helps the growth of good bacteria in the stomach.

The resistant starch content of green, unripe bananas is higher than that of ripe bananas, and they are also a good source of the dietary fiber pectin. Both of these have been connected to numerous health advantages, such as enhanced blood sugar regulation and intestinal health.

Meanwhile, ripe bananas are fantastic sources of quickly absorbed carbohydrates, making them ideal for refueling before exercise.

Oranges

Oranges are renowned for having a high vitamin C concentration; one orange contains 91% of the DV. They are also rich in fiber, plant polyphenols, potassium, folate, and thiamine (vitamin B1).
Consuming whole oranges may reduce levels of inflammation, blood pressure, cholesterol, and post-meal blood sugar, according to studies.

Despite having a large amount of minerals and antioxidants, 100% orange juice typically lacks dietary fiber. Choose juices with pulp over juices without because they do include some fiber.

However, try to consume oranges whole more frequently, and limit your intake of juice to no more than 1 cup (235 mL) every serving.

Dragon Fruit

The dragon fruit, often referred to as pitaya or pitahaya, is loaded with vitamins C and E, iron, fiber, and other nutrients. Additionally, it's a fantastic source of carotenoids including lycopene and beta-carotene.

For hundreds of years, people in Southeast Asian civilizations have valued dragon fruit as a fruit that promotes health. In Western nations, it has become more well-liked in recent decades.

Pomegranate

Pomegranates are well known for having a lot of antioxidants.

They include a long number of advantageous plant substances like flavonoids, tannins, and lignans. These battle free radicals and lower your chance of developing chronic diseases because of their potent antioxidant and anti-inflammatory capabilities.

8.5 ounces (250 mL) of pomegranate juice consumed daily for 12 weeks resulted in significantly lower levels of inflammation, according to a high-quality study, when compared to a placebo.

Guava
A great source of vitamin C is guava. In actuality, one fruit (55 grams) offers 140% of the daily value (DV) for this nutrient.

Additionally, when compared to other lycopene-rich foods like tomatoes, watermelon, and grapefruit, guava has some of the greatest concentrations.

Peaches
Another summertime favorite is peaches. They contain fiber, potassium, and vitamins A, C, and

E in good amounts. The carotenoids lutein, zeaxanthin, and beta-carotene are also present.

Both the flesh and the skin are nutritious, but the skin has a higher concentration of antioxidants that can assist your body fight free radicals. To get the most health advantages from peaches, eat the skin as well.

Fortunately, peaches appear to have identical nutritional value whether you eat them fresh or canned. But if you decide to buy peaches in a can, be sure they are packed in water rather than sweet syrup.

Kiwi

Kiwi, also referred to as the Chinese gooseberry, is very beneficial to your health.

It is an excellent source of fiber, potassium, folate, and vitamin E and is high in vitamin C. The carotenoids lutein, zeaxanthin, and beta carotene, which promote eye health and become more prevalent as fruits ripen, are also abundant in it.

Additionally, it has been utilized for hundreds of years in traditional Chinese medicine to assist digestion and intestinal health.

Its soluble and insoluble fiber, polyphenols, and digestive enzymes like actinidin are responsible for these advantages.

Consuming two kiwis per day for three days increased stool frequency and softened stool, according to small research, suggesting it may help cure moderate constipation

Olives

Olives are a fantastic complement to your diet, even though you might not immediately think of them as fruit.

They are a great source of copper, oleic acid, and vitamin E, all monounsaturated fatty acids.

They contain a lot of plant polyphenols, including quercetin, hydroxytyrosol, and oleuropein, which have antioxidant and anti-inflammatory activities.

In reality, a substantial portion of the Mediterranean diet includes whole olives and olive oil, which may reduce the risk of heart disease, type 2 diabetes, cognitive decline, overweight, and obesity, according to research.

The conclusion
Numerous tasty and healthy fruits can promote good health.

There are many other fruits you can choose from, even though this list only includes 10 of the healthiest fruits.

Make sure to consume a range of vibrant fruits every day to get the most advantages.

Chapter 3. Vegetables

A variety of edible plants called vegetables are generally eaten as a part of a balanced diet. They frequently stand out for having few calories, a lot of fiber, and a variety of vital nutrients like vitamins, minerals, and antioxidants. You can eat vegetables in a variety of ways, such as raw, cooked, steamed, roasted, or juiced.

Typical illustrations of veggies include:
Leafy greens: Arugula, Swiss chard, lettuce, spinach, and other varieties.
Broccoli, cauliflower, cabbage, Brussels sprouts, and bok choy are examples of cruciferous vegetables.
Carrots, potatoes, sweet potatoes, beets, and radishes are examples of root vegetables.

Alliums include leeks, shallots, garlic, and onions.

Nightshades include potatoes (even though they are a tuber), bell peppers, eggplant, and tomatoes.

Green beans, peas, lentils, chickpeas, and soybeans are examples of legumes.

Zucchini, butternut, acorn, and pumpkin are all types of squash.

Melons and cucumbers: cantaloupes, honeydews, watermelons, and cucumbers.

Asparagus, mushrooms, maize, artichokes, and okra are among the extras.

Due to their high nutritious content, vegetables offer a variety of health advantages. They are a great source of dietary fiber, which promotes good weight management and aids in digestion.

Additionally, they include vital nutrients like vitamin C, vitamin A, potassium, and folate. Regular vegetable consumption is linked to a lower risk of chronic illnesses like heart disease, several malignancies, and obesity.

It's crucial to remember that some items, like tomatoes, avocados, and olives, are technically considered to be fruits by botanical standards but are frequently used and consumed as vegetables in culinary contexts.

Chapter 4. Juicing And Weight Loss

Some people use the well-liked approach of juicing as part of their weight loss program. To make the juice drink, the liquid from fruits and vegetables must be extracted. Juicing is frequently marketed as a means to cleanse the body, up your vitamin intake, and maybe even help you lose weight.

Even though juicing can be a practical way to consume a variety of fruits and vegetables, it's vital to proceed with caution, especially if weight loss is your primary objective. Considering the following will help:

Juices can include a lot of natural sugars and calories, especially if they are mostly made of fruits. Fruits are healthy and contain fiber, however, juicing concentrates the sugars by removing the majority of the fiber. Without offering the same amount of satisfaction as whole fruits or vegetables, this can increase calorie intake.

Nutrient Balance: To create a balanced nutrient profile, make sure your juicing recipes use a range of fruits and vegetables. Leafy greens, vegetables, and low-sugar fruits can be added to your juices to increase the variety of nutrients and lessen the effect on blood sugar levels.

Satisfaction and Sustainability: Juicing can be a helpful technique to supplement a healthy diet, but depending only on juices for a lengthy period may leave you deficient in key nutrients and leaving you feeling unfulfilled. Whole foods, such as fresh produce, lean meats, whole grains, and unsaturated fats, supply necessary fiber and encourage satiety.

Juices can be nutrient-dense, but they are not a miracle cure for weight loss, according to metabolism and weight loss. A balanced diet, frequent exercise, and alterations to one's lifestyle are often necessary for long-term weight loss. Instead than concentrating on quick remedies, it's crucial to develop long-term behaviors.

Consultation with a Healthcare Professional: It's important to speak with a healthcare professional before making any big dietary changes, including juicing, if you have any underlying medical concerns like diabetes or digestive disorders or if you're taking medication.

In conclusion, juicing can be a beneficial supplement to your diet when practiced in moderation and as a part of a varied, balanced diet. The sustainability of your weight loss efforts over the long term, as well as your overall calorie intake and nutrient balance, should be taken into consideration. Always seek tailored guidance based on your unique needs and objectives from a healthcare practitioner or a licensed dietitian.

Fruit-based juice recipes

Easy Apple Celery Juice:

A healthful beverage, apple, and celery juice is simple to make. A stimulating beverage with nutritional benefits is created by mixing sweet and sour components.

Due to its high polyphenol content, apple juice may lower the risk of heart attacks.
According to one investigation, it prevents LDL oxidation. Lipid and protein oxidation occurs before the breakdown of cholesterol to form oxidized cholesterol.

The risk of atherosclerosis and high blood pressure increases as cholesterol deposits build up on the arterial walls. Apple juice could help prevent this and improve the condition of your heart.

Lowers Blood Pressure
Celery juice has a remarkable nutritional profile as well. Electrolytes and vitamins A, C, and K are abundant in it.

Additionally, it possesses hypotensive qualities. A 2019 study found that giving celery juice to hypertensive patients significantly lowered their blood pressure.
It even turned out to be more successful than a low-sodium diet. Therefore, occasionally sipping celery juice may be a wise move to reduce the risk of hypertension.

Ingredients: Apple, both red and green
Minty celery and lemon juice
Sugar

INSTRUCTIONS

1 Rinse fruits and vegetables. Flow freely.

2 Cut apple slices from the core. To obtain apple juice, put apple slices through a juicer.

3 To obtain clear juice, pour apple juice through a fine-mesh strainer.

4. To obtain celery juice, run celery through the juicer. Apple juice, celery juice, lemon juice, and sugar should all be combined in a pitcher. Until the sugar melts, stir.

5. Over ice, pour the beverage into 4 glasses. Leafy mint is a nice garnish. Serve.

Improved exercise performance: It has been demonstrated that nitrates in beets improve endurance and athletic performance. Before exercising, drinking blueberry beet juice may increase blood flow, oxygen supply to muscles, and total exercise capability.

Blueberries are referred to as "brain berries" because of their potential cognitive advantages. The antioxidants in blueberries may lessen age-related cognitive loss and shield the brain from oxidative stress.

Beets' high dietary fiber content helps to support a healthy digestive system and regular bowel motions. A healthy digestive tract may be supported by consuming beet juice.

Blueberries and beets are nutrient-dense foods that are loaded with important vitamins and minerals. Beets are high in folate, potassium, and iron, while blueberries are a wonderful source of vitamin C, vitamin K, and manganese. Juice made from blueberries and beets can assist you in getting the nutrients you need.

Recipe

You'll need the following supplies and tools to make blueberry beet juice:

Ingredients:

Blueberries, 1 cup
a single little beet

1 to 2 cups of water, depending on the desired
consistency
(Optional, to taste) Sweetener
Ice cubes, if desired

Equipment:

Juicer or blender
Knife
chopping block
(Optional) Fine mesh strainer or cheesecloth
The following steps will show you how to make
blueberry beet juice:

To get rid of any dirt or debris, properly wash the
blueberries and beet.

For simpler blending or juicing, use a knife to peel
the beet and cut it into small bits or slices.

Put the beet and blueberries in a juicer or blender.

To the juicer or blender, add water. Depending on
how thick or thin you want your juice, start with 1
cup and modify the amount.

The ingredients should be juiced or blended until a smooth consistency is reached. If using a blender, run it for 1-2 minutes, or until the mixture is smooth and well blended. Follow the manufacturer's instructions if using a juicer.

Use a fine mesh strainer or cheesecloth to filter the mixture for a juice that is smoother and pulp-free. If you prefer the pulpy juice texture, you can skip this step.

If desired, add sweetener after tasting the juice. You can use your favorite sweeteners, such as honey, maple syrup, or another. Start with a little quantity and gradually increase it to the desired sweetness.

To uniformly distribute the sweetener, stir the liquid.

If preferred, pour the blueberry beet juice over ice cubes to create a cool, refreshing drink.

Juice should be poured into glasses and consumed right away. Fresh consumption of blueberry beet juice is recommended to maintain both its nutritious value and beautiful color.

Keep in mind that the size and freshness of the beet might affect how strong the flavor is. You are welcome to change the ratios to suit your tastes.

Fruit Juice Mix

Benefits

Tutti frutti juice is a delectable beverage that blends a variety of fruits to make a delightful concoction. Here are some potential advantages of consuming tutti frutti juice, though the precise advantages may differ depending on the fruits used in the juice:

Contains a variety of critical nutrients, including vitamins, minerals, and antioxidants. Tutti frutti juice is often produced from a variety of fruits. The immune system, general health, and several biological functions depend on these nutrients.

Water and fruit extracts make up the majority of tutti frutti juice, which makes it a good source of hydration. Maintaining physical processes, controlling body temperature, and sustaining general health all depend on staying appropriately hydrated.

Many of the fruits used to make tutti frutti juice are high in antioxidants, which aid in defending the body against dangerous free radicals. Antioxidants can maintain cellular health, lessen the risk of chronic illnesses, and minimize oxidative stress.

Digestive health: Bromelain and papain, two digestive enzymes, are present in some fruits included in tutti frutti juice, including pineapple and papaya. These enzymes can facilitate the breakdown of proteins and enhance nutrient absorption as well as general digestion.

Support for the immune system: Fruits high in vitamin C, such as oranges, strawberries, and kiwis, are frequently found in tutti frutti juice. It is well known that vitamin C supports collagen formation, immunological function, and antioxidant activity.

Fiber Content: Fruits like apples and berries, which are used to make tutti frutti juice, are high in dietary fiber. Fiber assists with digestion, encourages fullness, and supports regular bowel motions.

Energy increase: Fruits' natural sugars can provide you with a rapid, all-natural energy boost. Tutti frutti juice might aid in replenishing your body's glycogen reserves, giving you a source of energy for when you're exercising or just need a boost.

Though tutti frutti juice may have certain advantages, it's still best to eat it in moderation as part of a healthy diet. When choosing the fruits for your juice blend, keep in mind any unique dietary limitations or allergies you may have.

Recipe
The following is a recipe for a cool tutti frutti juice:

Ingredients:

1 cup of watermelon dice
1 cup of pineapple dice
1 cup of mango dice
1 cup of papaya, diced
1 cup of strawberries, chopped
Orange juice, 1 cup
one teaspoon of lemon juice
Ice cubes, if desired

Instructions:

1. All fruits should be washed and prepared by having the core, skin, and any necessary seeds removed. Cut them up into little bits.
2. Watermelon, pineapple, mango, papaya, and strawberries, all chopped, should be added to a blender.
3. Fruits should be blended until well-combined and smooth.
4. To get rid of any pulp or seeds, strain the fruit puree through a cheesecloth or fine-mesh strainer.
5. Refill the blender with the fruit juice that has been strained.
6. To fully integrate the flavors, add the orange juice and lemon juice to the blender and blend for an additional 20 to 30 seconds.
7. Depending on your preferences, add extra orange or lemon juice after tasting the juice to change its sweetness or sharpness.
8. If desired, include some ice cubes in the blender and blend until the juice is cold and foamy.
9. Pour the tutti frutti juice into glasses as soon as it's done and serve right away.

10. Enjoy your tutti frutti juice; it's refreshing!

Gazpacho Juice With Mango

Benefits

Mango gazpacho juice mixes the flavors of ripe mangoes with the conventional components of gazpacho, such as tomatoes, cucumbers, and herbs, to create a revitalizing and wholesome beverage. Here are some potential health advantages of mango gazpacho juice, though the precise advantages may change based on the precise recipe and components used:

High in nutrients: Mangoes are a great source of potassium, vitamin C, vitamin A, and other vital vitamins and minerals. Lycopene, an antioxidant that may help prevent some types of cancer, is found in abundance in tomatoes. Water-retaining cucumbers also contain vitamins K and C.

Mangoes and tomatoes are both abundant in antioxidants, which can aid in defending the body's cells from damage brought on by free radicals. Chronic disorders like heart disease and some forms of cancer are related to a lower probability of developing antioxidants.

Hydration: Because of its high water content, gazpacho juice, notably mango gazpacho, is a hydrating beverage. To maintain healthy digestion, food absorption, and temperature regulation, it is crucial to stay hydrated.

Support for the digestive system: Gazpacho juice contains a considerable level of dietary fiber because of the inclusion of mangoes, tomatoes, and cucumbers. Constipation is avoided and a healthy gut is supported by fiber, which also aids in proper digestion.

Support for the immune system: Citrus fruits, including mangoes, are recognized for having high vitamin C content, which is necessary for a robust immune system. Vitamin C stimulates the synthesis of collagen, a protein crucial for healthy skin and joints, and aids in wound healing and infection prevention.

Weight management: Gazpacho juice is a nutrient-dense, low-calorie solution that is a good choice for people who are controlling their weight. The presence of fiber may aid in promoting satiety and lessen the likelihood of overeating.

The advantages listed are broad, thus it's crucial to keep in mind that individual outcomes may differ. Before making big changes to your diet, it's also a good idea to speak with a healthcare provider or trained dietitian if you have any particular health issues or illnesses.

Recipe

The following is the recipe for mango gazpacho juice:

Ingredients:

Pitted and peeled two ripe mangos
Peeled and seeded one medium cucumber
1 seeded red bell pepper
one little red onion
2 garlic cloves
1 seeded jalapeno pepper, optionally for heat
2 teaspoons of lime juice, fresh
14 cups fresh leaves of cilantro

Fresh mint leaves, 1/4 cup
pepper and salt as desired
(Optional) Ice cubes for cooling

Instructions:

1. Mangoes, cucumbers, bell peppers, red onions, garlic, and jalapenos (if using) should all be finely chopped before being added to a blender or food processor.
2. Fresh lime juice, cilantro, and mint leaves should all be added to the mixer.
3. Blend each component until it is smooth and evenly distributed. If you want cooled gazpacho juice, you can add a few ice cubes.
4. As desired, add salt and pepper to the mixture **Juice Made From Vegetables**.
5. Fill glasses or a pitcher with the gazpacho fluid.
6. The gazpacho juice can be served right away or chilled for a couple of hours to let the flavors merge.
7. If preferred, add more cilantro leaves or a slice of lime to the mango gazpacho fluid before serving.

Enjoy your juice made with cool mango gazpacho!

4. Pineapple Kiwi Juice

Benefits

A delightful and refreshing concoction, kiwi pineapple juice has several possible health advantages. The following are some advantages of drinking kiwi pineapple juice:

Rich in vitamins and minerals: Both kiwis and pineapple are first-rate suppliers of these nutrients. Kiwis are particularly well-known for their high vitamin C content, which works as an antioxidant, immune system booster, and promoter of collagen synthesis. Bromelain is an enzyme blend found in pineapples that helps with digestion and has anti-inflammatory qualities. Both fruits also include potassium, vitamins A and E, and other nutrients.

Bromelain, an enzyme found in pineapple that helps digestion by dissolving proteins and enhancing nutrient absorption, is also good for the digestive system. Constipation, bloating, and indigestion symptoms can all be helped by it. Kiwi, on the other hand, has fiber that helps healthy digestion and encourages regular bowel motions.

Kiwi and pineapple both have anti-inflammatory qualities as a result of the presence of numerous bioactive components. This may be beneficial for treating diseases like inflammatory bowel disease, gout, and arthritis by reducing inflammation in the body.

Vitamin C, vitamin E, and other phytochemicals are among the many antioxidants found in kiwi and pineapple. When free radicals are neutralized in the body, oxidative stress is reduced, which may lower the chance of developing chronic illnesses including heart disease and some types of cancer.

Support for the immune system: Vitamin C, which is essential for a strong immune system, is abundant in kiwis. Along with other immune-boosting elements like bromelain, pineapple also includes vitamin C. Kiwi pineapple juice can enhance overall well-being by boosting the immune system when consumed regularly.

Kiwi pineapple juice is a hydrating beverage since both kiwis and pineapples are high in water content. Numerous biological processes depend on optimal hydration, which also supports good skin, sound digestion, and overall well-being.

Although kiwi pineapple juice may have some health advantages, it's still best to eat it in moderation as part of a healthy diet. It's important to keep in mind that everyone reacts to food differently, so if you have any particular dietary problems or conditions, it's better to listen to your body and seek medical advice.

Recipe

An easy recipe for Kiwi Pineapple Juice is provided below:

Ingredients:

2 mature kiwis
1 cup of chunks of fresh pineapple
one water cup
Ice cubes, if desired

Instructions:

1. Kiwis should be peeled and sliced into small pieces.
2. Slice up the pineapple, removing the rough core.
3. Blend the pineapple and kiwi chunks in a blender.
4. the blender with water.
5. Blend the ingredients collectively and smoothly.
6. If ice is wanted, add it to the blender and reblend to chill it.
7. Juice is poured into glasses.
8. Kiwi pineapple juice should be served right away.
9. Depending on your preferred level of sweetness, you can change the amount of kiwi and pineapple. Additionally, you can blend in a tablespoon or two of honey or another sweetener of your choosing if you want a sweeter juice. You are welcome to experiment and adjust the recipe to your preferences. Take pleasure in your hydrating Kiwi Pineapple juice!

Mango-Melon Juice

Benefits

Mango melon juice combines the flavors and health advantages of both mangoes and melons into one energizing and nourishing beverage. The following are some advantages of drinking mango melon juice:

Mangoes and melons are both excellent providers of vitamins and minerals that are needed for good health. Melons are high in vitamin A, vitamin C, potassium, and antioxidants, whereas mangoes are high in vitamin C, vitamin A, and folate. Mango melon juice is a great way to increase your consumption of these vital nutrients.

Mangoes and melons both have a lot of water, making them excellent for staying hydrated. Mango melon juice can be particularly helpful when it's hot outside or after exercise when your body needs to replace fluids.

The antioxidants beta-carotene, lutein, and zeaxanthin can be found in mangoes and melons.

These substances may lessen the chance of developing chronic diseases by assisting the body's defense mechanisms against dangerous free radicals and shielding cells from oxidative stress.

Foods high in dietary fiber, such as mangoes and melons, can aid in a healthy digestive system and ward off constipation. Juice from a mango melon can help you have regular bowel movements and enhance your overall digestive health.

Support for the immune system: The vitamin C in melons and mangoes can fortify the immune system and aid in its correct operation. Mango melon juice regularly may help guard against infections and common diseases.

Skin health: Mangoes and melons have significant levels of vitamin C and other antioxidants, which help to maintain healthy skin. These nutrients aid in the development of collagen, which can increase skin suppleness and lessen the visibility of wrinkles.

Weight loss: Mango melon juice has a high water and fiber content while having a comparatively low calorie and fat level. By encouraging satiety and lowering caloric intake, including this juice in a balanced diet may aid in weight management.

Keep in mind that mango melon juice should only be used as a part of a varied and balanced diet, even though it may have certain health benefits. Additionally, individual outcomes may differ, so it's always a good idea to seek professional medical advice or nutrition guidance.

Recipe

An easy recipe for mango melon juice is provided below:

Ingredients:

one ripe mango
1 ripe melon, such as honeydew or cantaloupe
Cold water, 1 cup
Ice cubes, if desired
(Optional and according to taste)

Instructions:

1. Prepare the fruits first. After peeling, separate the mango's flesh from the pit.
2. Mango should be cut into pieces and kept aside.
3. Scoop out the seeds after halving the melon. Cut the melon into cubes and remove the rind as well.
4. Juice the mango and melon chunks or put them in a blender.
5. To the juicer or blender, add the cold water.
6. Fruits should be juiced or blended until they are smooth. If using a blender, run it for one or two minutes at high speed. Follow the manufacturer's instructions if using a juicer.
7. After tasting the juice, you can add sugar or honey to sweeten it if you like. Start with a little and then increase or decrease as desired.
8. You may either pour your juice over ice or add a few ice cubes to the blender if you want it chilly.
9. Pour the juice into glasses as soon as it's done and serve right away.
10. Take a sip of your cool mango melon juice.

6. Juice With Strawberry Lemonade

Benefits

A revitalizing drink that mixes the tartness of lemons with the sweetness of strawberries is strawberry lemonade juice. Due to the natural qualities of its ingredients, it not only tastes good but also may have certain health benefits. The following are a few possible advantages of strawberry lemonade juice:

Rich in vitamin C: The potent antioxidant vitamin C can be found in a variety of foods, including strawberries and lemons. Vitamin C works as an antioxidant to prevent cell damage from free radicals, boosts the immune system, and encourages collagen synthesis for healthy skin.

Strawberries include a variety of antioxidants, including anthocyanins, ellagic acid, and quercetin. Lemons also include flavonoids and vitamin C, which are antioxidants. These antioxidants assist the body in scavenging free radicals, which can lower the risk of chronic illnesses and improve general health.

Staying hydrated is essential for preserving general health and well-being. Strawberry lemonade juice is a tasty method to up your hydration consumption, especially when it's hot outside or you're exercising.

Heart health: Lemons and strawberries both contain substances that may be good for the heart. Strawberries are a great source of anthocyanins, a type of flavonoid that has been linked to a lower risk of heart disease. Hesperidin, a flavonoid found in lemons, may help lower blood pressure and lessen inflammation, promoting heart health.

Lemons are renowned for their advantages to the digestive system. Lemon juice's acidity can promote the formation of digestive juices, which helps with digestion. Strawberries also include a lot of dietary fiber, which helps maintain regular bowel movements and a healthy digestive tract.

Enhanced energy: Strawberries' natural sugars might give you a rapid energy boost, and the vitamin

C in lemons and strawberries may help you fight weariness and have more energy.

Weight loss: Strawberry lemonade juice might be a more wholesome substitute for sweetened beverages and sodas. You may sate your want for something sweet by choosing this energizing beverage without ingesting too many calories or artificial ingredients.

Although strawberry lemonade juice might provide many advantages, it's crucial to remember that moderation is the key. A healthcare practitioner or nutritionist can offer you individualized guidance about your diet and any particular health issues you may have.

Recipe

Here is a quick recipe for a tasty strawberry lemonade:

Ingredients:

1 cup of strawberries, fresh
4 to 6 lemons
1/2 cup sugar, taste-tested

Water in 4 glasses
An ice cube
You can utilize fresh mint leaves as a garnish.

Instructions:

1. Strawberry stalks should be removed after washing. To make mixing simpler, cut them into smaller pieces.
2. To obtain the juice from the lemons, juice them. You can use either an electric or a manual juicer.
3. Sliced strawberries should be added to a blender and blended until smooth.
4. To get rid of any seeds or pulp, pass the strawberry puree through a fine-mesh sieve. About 1 cup of strawberry juice should be consumed.
5. Combine the strawberry juice, lemon juice, sugar, and water in a pitcher.
6. until the sugar melts, vigorously stir. Taste it and, if necessary, add additional sugar or lemon juice to change the sweetness or sharpness.

7. To allow the flavors to mingle, chill the strawberry lemonade in the fridge for at least an hour.
8. When it's time to serve, put ice cubes in glasses and then pour the chilled strawberry lemonade over them.
9. For an optional freshness and scent boost, garnish each glass with a few fresh mint leaves.

Enjoy your homemade strawberry lemonade juice after a quick stir!

You are welcome to change the amount of sweetness or bitterness to suit your tastes.

For a bubbly twist, you can also try adding a tiny bit of sparkling water or soda. Enjoy!

Fruit Mint Blast

Benefits

Berry mint blast juice mixes the flavors of berries and mint to create a revitalizing and wholesome beverage. Here are some potential advantages of ingesting berry mint blast juice, albeit the precise advantages may differ based on the ingredients and cooking technique:

Berries that are high in antioxidants include blueberries, strawberries, and raspberries. Antioxidants aid in defending your body against oxidative stress, which can lead to cellular damage and chronic diseases.

Support for the Immune System: Berries are well-known for having a lot of vitamin C, which is important for a strong immune system. Additionally, mint has a few substances that could help the immune system.

Juices can help you stay hydrated by adding to your daily fluid intake, especially if you have trouble getting enough water in. It's critical to drink enough water to preserve general health and well-being.

Berries are rich in nutrients, including fiber, vitamins, and minerals. Numerous minerals, including vitamin C, vitamin K, manganese, and folate, can be found in them.

Digestive Health: Mint has long been used as a digestive aid. It might lessen bloating, ease digestive discomfort, and encourage regular bowel motions. Berries and mint together can produce a flavor that is both revitalizing and refreshing, making it a tasty beverage choice. Berries' natural sugars might also give you a rapid energy boost.

Weight loss: Berries' low calorie and high fiber content can help you feel fuller for longer and support your weight loss objectives.

It's important to keep in mind that the overall advantages of any juice can change based on the precise ingredients, the amounts ingested, and the person's general diet and health. Berry mint blast juice can be a healthy complement to a balanced diet, but it's crucial to use moderation and lead a healthy lifestyle in general when consuming it.

Recipe

The Berry Mint Blast juice is a tasty beverage that mixes the freshness of fresh mint with the sweetness of berries. Here is a straightforward recipe for making Berry Mint Blast juice at home:

Ingredients:

1 cup of mixed berries, including raspberries, blueberries, and strawberries
5 or 6 new leaves of mint
one water cup
1 tablespoon of your preferred sweetener, such as honey
Ice cubes, if desired

Instructions:

1. Thoroughly wash the berries and take off any stems or leaves.
2. Put the berries and mint leaves in a food processor or blender.
3. Water should be added to the blender, then the mixture should be blended on high speed until it is well incorporated and smooth.

4. If desired, add honey or another sweetener of your choice to the juice after tasting it to increase its sweetness.
5. To include the sweetener, blend once more.
6. A few ice cubes can be added to the blender and blended with the juice if you would like a cooler beverage.
7. Pour the juice into glasses once it has been mixed to the correct consistency.
8. You might choose to add some more berries or a sprig of fresh mint to the juice's garnish.
9. I'm done now! You can now enjoy your cool Berry Mint Blast juice.

To have the greatest flavor and texture, serve it right away.

Strawberry Banana Juice With Cilantro

Benefits

Cilantro and Strawberry Banana Juice have several health advantages. The important vitamins, minerals, and antioxidants found in strawberries and bananas assist digestion, the immune system, and heart health. The leaves of cilantro, also known as coriander, offer extra nutrients and may have anti-inflammatory and antioxidant qualities. It's important to keep in mind that individual advantages may differ and that a balanced diet consisting of a variety of fruits and vegetables is necessary for general well-being.

Recipe
An easy recipe for strawberry banana juice with cilantro is provided below:

Ingredients:

1 cup fresh or frozen strawberries
two ripe bananas
14 cups fresh leaves of cilantro
one water cup
Ice cubes, if desired
Sweetener or honey (optional, if desired)

Instructions:

1. Thoroughly clean the cilantro leaves and strawberries. For simpler blending, peel the bananas and cut them into smaller pieces.
2. Strawberries, bananas, and cilantro leaves should all be placed in a blender.
3. If you want a cooler juice, pour in the water and optionally add ice cubes.
4. Blend the ingredients collectively and smoothly.
5. If necessary, add honey or your favorite sweetener after tasting the juice.
6. To include the sweetener, blend just once more.
7. Juice should be poured into glasses and served right away.
8. Take pleasure in your revitalizing Strawberry Banana Juice with a hint of cilantro!

9. Blended Strawberry Kiwi Juice

Benefits

In addition to being a great source of vitamins, antioxidants, and minerals from both fruits, blended strawberry kiwi juice has many other advantages.

Due to its high water content, it may help bolster immunity, support heart health, ease digestion, and offer hydration. Furthermore, the flavor profile that is produced by the blending of strawberries and kiwis is tasty and energizing. Always keep in mind that it's ideal to incorporate it into a balanced diet.

Recipe

Here is a straightforward recipe for a revitalizing strawberry-kiwi juice mix:

Ingredients:

1 cup hulled and cut strawberries
2 sliced and peeled kiwis
1 cup of iced water
1 tablespoon of your preferred sweetener, such as honey
Ice cubes, if desired

Instructions:

1. Put the kiwi slices and strawberries in a food processor or blender.
2. Fill the blender with cold water.

3. If more sweetness is required, you can add a spoonful of honey or another sweetener to the blender.
4. The mixture needs to be uniform and well-combined after being blended at high speed. To make sure all the fruit is blended, you might need to pause regularly and scrape down the sides of the blender.
5. Taste the mixture and, if necessary, add additional honey or water to change the sweetness or consistency.
6. If desired, add a few ice cubes to the blender and run it once more to chill and froth the liquid.
7. Pour the juice mixture into glasses after it reaches the appropriate consistency.
8. Enjoy your tart strawberry-kiwi juice combination right away!
9. To suit your personal preferences, feel free to change the quantities of strawberries, kiwis, or sweetness. If you want the juice to have a smoother texture, you can also strain it. Enjoy!

Ginger Orange Carrot Juice:

Benefits

Because of the combination of these healthy ingredients, orange carrot ginger juice offers several health advantages. Here are a few possible advantages:

Oranges are rich in vitamin C, which supports a healthy immune system and the ability to fend against illnesses. Beta-carotene, another mineral that strengthens the immune system, is found in carrots. Ginger's antibacterial qualities can help to stave off infections.

Antioxidant defense: Antioxidants like vitamin C and beta-carotene are abundant in oranges and carrots. These antioxidants assist in defending the body against oxidative stress brought on by free radicals, which can harm cells and exacerbate chronic illnesses.

Ginger includes a substance called gingerol, which has strong anti-inflammatory benefits. Regular ginger consumption may help the body's inflammation decrease, which is good for ailments including arthritis, inflammatory bowel disease, and overall pain brought on by inflammation.

Digestive support: Ginger has long been used to aid digestion. It can lessen bloating, ease nausea, and enhance digestion in general. Dietary fiber, which carrots provide an excellent amount of, helps maintain a healthy digestive system and regular bowel motions.

Heart health: Oranges are renowned for having high quantities of potassium and vitamin C, both of which are beneficial for the heart. Dietary fiber and antioxidants, both of which are found in carrots, have been linked to a lower risk of heart disease. Additionally, ginger may reduce blood pressure and enhance blood circulation.

Skin health: The antioxidants and vitamin C present in oranges and carrots can support the maintenance of healthy skin. These nutrients aid in the synthesis of collagen, which increases skin suppleness and aids in the preservation of a youthful appearance.

Acne and eczema may both benefit from ginger's anti-inflammatory effects.

While orange carrot ginger juice can have health advantages, it should be drunk as a supplement to a balanced diet rather than as the only source of nutrients. A healthcare expert should always be consulted for specific advice because individual outcomes may differ.

Recipe

An easy recipe for orange carrot ginger juice is provided below:

Ingredients:

4 big carrots
two oranges.
Piece of ginger, 1 inch long

Instructions:

1. Thoroughly wash the ginger, oranges, and carrots.

2. Use a knife or a vegetable peeler to remove the carrot and ginger skin.
3. To make the carrots and ginger easier to juice, cut them into smaller pieces.
4. To get fresh orange juice, cut the oranges in half and squeeze out the juice.
5. Juice the carrot slices and ginger after adding them to a juicer.
6. When the carrot and ginger juice is finished, put it in a jug or pitcher with the freshly squeezed orange juice.
7. To make sure the flavors are dispersed equally, stir thoroughly.
8. If you want the juice to have a smoother texture, you can, but are not required to, strain it through a fine-mesh sieve.
9. Orange carrot ginger juice can be chilled for later use or served right away over ice.

Note: You can change the amounts of ginger, oranges, and carrots to suit your taste. You are welcome to experiment and adjust the amount of each item to your desire.

Take pleasure in your hydrating and nourishing orange carrot ginger juice!

Juice of Pine-Lav

Benefits

The tropical sweetness of pineapple is combined with the aromatic and relaxing qualities of lavender to create the delectable and delightful drink known as pineapple lavender juice. While the precise advantages of this juice combination may differ depending on personal tastes and health situations, the following are some possible advantages linked to its main ingredients:

Pineapple has a high vitamin content, particularly vitamin C, as well as minerals including manganese and the digestive enzyme bromelain. Although ingested in modest doses, lavender contains several phytochemicals, antioxidants, and essential oils.

Digestive Aid: The pineapple compound bromelain is well-known for its ability to aid in digestion. It aids in the breakdown of proteins, supports digestion, and may lessen bloating or indigestion.

Anti-Inflammatory Effects: Lavender and pineapple both have anti-inflammatory effects. Bromelain, a chemical found in pineapple, may aid to lessen inflammation in the body, and linalool and linalyl acetate, found in lavender, have anti-inflammatory properties.

Support for antioxidants: Both pineapple and lavender are abundant in antioxidants that assist in defending cells against oxidative stress and harm brought on by free radicals. Antioxidants are important for overall health and may lower the chance of developing chronic illnesses.

Lavender is well known for its relaxing effects. It also relieves stress. Being calming, lavender is well-recognized and has stress-relieving properties. Juice made from lavender may aid in promoting relaxation and calmness.

Hydration: Pineapple lavender juice can be a cool, hydrating beverage, particularly in hot weather or after exercise. A healthy body requires adequate hydration to support many biological processes.

It's important to keep in mind that everyone reacts differently to certain foods and drinks, and some people can be allergic or sensitive to certain foods like pineapple or lavender. Before making any dietary changes, it is always a good idea to speak with a healthcare provider if you have any health issues or special dietary needs.

Recipe

A recipe for pineapple lavender juice is provided below:

Ingredients:

1 ripe pineapple, one
1 tablespoon of lavender flowers, dried
Water in 4 glasses
1-2 teaspoons of honey or other preferred sweetener
Ice cubes, if desired

Instructions:

1. The pineapple should be peeled, cored, and cut into pieces.
2. the water will be boiled in a saucepan.

3. The dried lavender flowers should be added to the boiling water and simmered for five minutes.
4. After turning off the heat, let the water that has been infused with lavender cool for a while.
5. Make use of cheesecloth or a fine-mesh strainer to remove the lavender flowers from the liquid.
6. The pineapple chunks and the water flavored with lavender should be blended.
7. Blend the ingredients well and smoothly.
8. If desired, add honey or another sweetener after tasting the juice. To suit your tastes, adjust the sweetness.
9. To get rid of any leftover fibers or particles, you can pass the juice through a fine-mesh strainer if you choose.
10. For at least one hour, refrigerate the juice.
11. If desired, pour the pineapple lavender juice over ice cubes.
12. Add a wedge of pineapple or an optional sprig of fresh lavender as a garnish.
13. Take pleasure in your energizing pineapple lavender juice!

Note: You can slightly increase the number of dried lavender flowers if you desire a stronger lavender flavor. But take care not to overwhelm the pineapple flavor.

Blended Papaya And Pineapple Juice

Benefits

Due to the pairing of these two fruits, papaya pineapple juice blend may provide several advantages. The following are some potential advantages of drinking a papaya-pineapple juice combination:

Digestive health: Papaya and pineapple both contain digestive enzymes. Pineapple contains bromelain, whereas papain is found in papaya. These enzymes may lessen bloating and indigestion by assisting in the breakdown of proteins and enhancing digestion in general.

Bromelain and papain are two substances found in pineapple and papaya that have anti-inflammatory properties. These substances could be useful in treating diseases including inflammatory bowel disease and arthritis by lowering inflammation in the body.

Support for the immune system: Papaya and pineapple are both great providers of vitamin C, which is necessary for a strong immune system. An increase in vitamin C from drinking papaya pineapple juice can aid to improve general health by boosting the immune system.

Vitamin C, beta-carotene, and flavonoids are just a few of the antioxidants found in papaya and pineapple. Antioxidants may have anti-aging properties and assist in defending the body against harm from dangerous free radicals.

Hydration and detoxification: A papaya pineapple juice blend is an electrolyte replenisher and hydrating beverage. Additionally, it can have modest diuretic qualities that increase urine production and support detoxification.

Papaya and pineapple are both nutrient-rich fruits that are loaded with important vitamins and minerals. A good source of potassium, vitamin E, folate, and vitamin A is papaya. Manganese, vitamin B6, and copper are abundant in pineapple. Drinking a drink made of papaya and pineapple can give you access to a variety of nutrients that are vital for good health.

Skin health: The papaya pineapple juice blend's rich vitamin C and antioxidant content helps support healthy skin. These vitamins and minerals might encourage the creation of collagen, guard against skin damage, and keep you looking young.

You should always eat a balanced diet that includes a range of fruits and vegetables because individual outcomes may vary. Before making any big dietary changes, it's also a good idea to speak with a healthcare provider if you have any particular health issues or medical illnesses.

Recipe

Here is a quick recipe for a cool papaya-pineapple juice combination:

Ingredients:

1 papaya, ripe
1 miniature pineapple
Cold water, 1 cup
Ice cubes, if desired
If desired, add honey or sugar for sweetness.

Instructions:

1. Peeling the papaya and taking out the seeds should come first. Slice it into pieces.
2. Cut the pineapple into chunks after peeling it and removing the core.
3. Blend the papaya and pineapple pieces in a food processor.
4. Blender with cold water added.
5. A spoonful or two of honey or sugar can be added here if you prefer a sweeter drink.
6. Until you get a juice that is smooth and well-combined, blend everything at high speed.
7. To get rid of any pulp or fibers, you can pass the juice through a fine mesh sieve if you'd like.

8. If using, pour the juice into glasses with ice cubes.

9. Enjoy your delightful papaya pineapple juice blend right away!

You are welcome to change the amount of sweetness or water to suit your tastes. If you'd like, you could also add a squeeze of lime juice for a zesty edge. Enjoy!

Apple Honeydew Juice

Benefits

Due to the honeydew melon and apple combination, honeydew apple juice is a tasty and healthy beverage that can provide several advantages. While there may not be much specific research on honeydew apple juice, we may talk about the possible advantages of the various components.

The water content in apples and honeydew melon is high, which can help with healthy hydration. To maintain healthy physical processes and general well-being, it's crucial to stay hydrated.

Rich in nutrients: Apples and honeydew melon both contain a lot of important vitamins, minerals, and antioxidants. Vitamins C and K, potassium, folate, and dietary fiber are all present in honeydew melon. Vitamin C, dietary fiber, antioxidants, and phytonutrients like quercetin are all present in apples.

Honeydew melon and apple together can offer a healthy dosage of antioxidants, which aid in the body's fight against free radicals. Antioxidants shield cells from oxidative stress, which can speed up aging and cause chronic diseases.

The health of the digestive system: Apples and honeydew melon both include dietary fiber, which facilitates digestion and encourages regular bowel movements. A healthy digestive system can be supported by getting enough fiber.

Support for the immune system: Apples and honeydew melon include vitamins and antioxidants that can help boost the immune system. Particular vitamin C is well known for strengthening the immune system.

Honeydew melon and apples are low in calories and high in fiber, which can help improve satiety and aid in weight management. A balanced diet that includes honeydew apple juice may help with weight loss goals.

Although honeydew apple juice can be a nourishing complement to a balanced diet, it's vital to keep in mind that it should only be consumed occasionally. Individual outcomes and advantages may also differ based on elements including general dietary habits, way of life, and medical issues.

Recipe

An easy recipe for honeydew apple juice is provided below:

Ingredients:

one large honeydew melon
two apples, preferably green
1 tablespoon of optionally additional lemon juice for extra tang

(Optional) Ice cubes for serving

Instructions:

1. Wash the apples and honeydew melon well.
2. Scoop out the seeds, remove the rind, and cut the honeydew melon in half. Slice up the melon's flesh into manageable pieces.
3. Apples should be cored and chopped into smaller pieces.
4. Apple and honeydew melon chunks should be placed in a blender.
5. Until the mixture is smooth, blend the components at a high speed. To get rid of any pulp or fibers, you can strain the juice using cheesecloth or a fine-mesh strainer.
6. Add a tablespoon of lemon juice and combine it with the mixture if you prefer a tangier flavor.
7. Once the juice has been mixed, taste it to check for sweetness or tartness. If necessary, add extra honeydew melon, apple, or lemon juice.
8. In a glass pitcher or into individual glasses, pour the juice.

9. For a cool refreshment, place ice cubes in the glasses, if preferred.

Enjoy your homemade honeydew apple juice right away!

You are welcome to play around with the ratios and change them to suit your personal preferences. If you want juice with a thinner consistency or to slightly diluted the juice, you can also add a dash of water. Take pleasure in your hydrating honeydew apple juice!

Cucumber-Melon Juice

Benefits

Cucumber melon juice has several potential advantages because it combines two hydrated and refreshing fruits. The following are some possible advantages of cucumber melon juice:

Cucumber and melon juice is a great way to stay hydrated because they both have high water content.

Maintaining healthy physiological processes and promoting general well-being requires adequate hydration.

Rich in nutrients: Melons and cucumbers are loaded with healthy vitamins, minerals, and antioxidants. Melons include vitamins A and C, potassium, and folate, while cucumbers are an excellent source of vitamin K, vitamin C, potassium, and magnesium.

Cucumber melon juice has antioxidants that can help shield your cells from damage brought on by dangerous chemicals known as free radicals. Antioxidants can improve general health and lower the risk of developing chronic illnesses.

Cucumbers are a good source of dietary fiber, which helps with digestion and encourages regular bowel movements. Melons' abundant water content and natural enzymes may also have a calming impact on the digestive system.

Weight loss: Due to its low calorie and high water content, cucumber melon juice might be a helpful complement to a weight loss regimen. Maybe you'll feel more content and full, which lowers your risk of overeating.

Cucumbers and melons are well-known for having beneficial effects on the skin. They have nutrients and antioxidants that can moisturize the skin, support healthy skin, and possibly even out complexion.

Due to its moisturizing and diuretic qualities, cucumber melon juice can serve as a natural detoxifier. It might support kidney function and aid in toxin removal from the body.

Although the advantages listed above are based on the general nutritional composition of cucumber and melon, individual experiences may differ. As with any food or drink, moderation is crucial. It's also a good idea to seek out individualized guidance from a healthcare provider or nutritionist whenever possible.

Recipe

An easy recipe for preparing cucumber melon juice is provided below:

Ingredients:

one medium cucumber
1 ripe melon, such as a cantaloupe or honeydew
Fresh mint leaves are an optional flavoring.
(Optional) Ice cubes for serving

Instructions:

1. Under running water, give the cucumber and melon a thorough wash.
2. Slice the cucumber in half lengthwise, and if preferred, remove the seeds. Depending on your preference, you can either keep the skin on or peel it.
3. Scoop out the flesh after cutting the melon in half and removing the seeds.
4. To make the cucumber and melon simpler to combine, chop them into smaller pieces.
5. Blend the cukes and slices of melon in a blender.
6. A few fresh mint leaves can be added to the blender if you'd like more taste. The amount of mint can be changed to suit your personal preferences.

7. The ingredients should be thoroughly blended to reach a creamy consistency. To aid in blending, you might if necessary add a little water.
8. After blending, filter the juice to get rid of any pulp or solids using a fine-mesh screen or cheesecloth. If you prefer a richer juice, omit this step.
9. If desired, place ice cubes in a glass with the cucumber melon juice.
10. Serve the juice cold after thoroughly stirring it.
11. You are welcome to change the amounts and ingredients to suit your tastes. To improve the flavor, you can try experimenting with adding additional fruits or veggies. Take a sip of your cooling cucumber melon juice.

Watermelon And Mango Juice

Benefits

Mango watermelon juice is a wonderful and revitalizing drink that combines the juicy and hydrating qualities of watermelon with the sweet and tropical flavors of mango. Here are some potential advantages of ingesting mango watermelon juice, though it's important to note that specific health benefits may differ depending on individual circumstances and general dietary intake:

Watermelon is well-known for having a high water content, which aids in maintaining your hydration. Mangoes also add to the juice's overall water content, making it a healthy option for rehydrating and quenching thirst.

Mangoes and watermelons are both nutrient-rich foods that are loaded with important vitamins and minerals. Mangoes are a fantastic source of potassium, folate, vitamin C, and vitamin A. Lycopene, vitamin A, vitamin C, and antioxidants are all abundant in watermelons.

Mangoes and watermelons are rich in antioxidants, which aid in defending the body against free radicals, unstable chemicals that can harm cells. Inflammation and oxidative stress are decreased by antioxidants, potentially improving general health.

An immune system booster, collagen formation, and wound healing all benefit from vitamin C, which can be found in mango watermelon juice.

Both mangoes and watermelons include dietary fiber, which helps with digestion and encourages regular bowel movements. Consuming foods high in fiber may help maintain a healthy digestive tract and prevent constipation.

Mangoes are a good source of vitamin A, which is necessary for healthy eyes and vision. Mango watermelon juice can help you get enough vitamin A if you drink it frequently.

Skin health: By boosting collagen production, guarding against free radical damage, and maintaining skin hydration, the vitamin C, antioxidants, and hydration included in mango watermelon juice may help to promote healthy skin.

It's crucial to remember that even though mango watermelon juice may have certain health advantages, a balanced diet should still include it and it shouldn't take the place of complete fruits and vegetables. Furthermore, since fruit juices can contain a lot of natural sugars, moderation is essential.

Recipe

An easy recipe for mango watermelon juice is provided below:

Ingredients:

2 cups of seedless sliced watermelon
1 mango, diced after being peeled
a teaspoon of lime juice
1-2 tablespoons of optional, taste-tested honey or sugar
Ice cubes, if desired

Instructions:

1. Prepare the mango and watermelon first. If necessary, remove the watermelon seeds before chopping them up. Mangoes should be peeled and diced as well.
2. Put the mango and watermelon cubes into a food processor or blender.

3. One lime juice should be squeezed into the blender. Lime juice gives the dish a wonderful acidic flavor that goes well with the fruits' sweetness.
4. You can add honey or sugar to your juice according to taste if you'd like it to be sweeter. Start with 1 tablespoon, then titrate to your taste.
5. Blend each component until it is smooth and evenly distributed. You can add water or ice cubes to the blender to achieve the desired consistency.
6. Juice should be poured into a glass after blending. If you want the juice to have a smoother texture, you can, but are not required to, strain it through a fine-mesh sieve.
7. You can choose to decorate the glass with a mint sprig or a slice of watermelon.
8. Enjoy the mango watermelon juice's cooling flavor right away!

You are welcome to change the ingredients and amounts to suit your tastes. savor the mango watermelon juice you produced at home!

Orange-kiwi juice

Benefits

Kiwi orange juice, which is produced by mixing orange juice and kiwi fruit, may have various health advantages. The following are some advantages of drinking kiwi orange juice:

Boost Your Vitamin C: Kiwis and oranges are both great sources of vitamin C. Even more vitamin C is found in kiwi fruit than in oranges. Vitamin C is an effective antioxidant that supports overall immunological health, boosts collagen production for good skin, and helps the body absorb iron.

Powerful antioxidants include vitamin C, which is abundant in kiwis and oranges and aids in the body's ability to combat dangerous free radicals. Antioxidants are essential for lowering oxidative stress and safeguarding the body from chronic illnesses.

The high fiber content of kiwi fruit is well-known for promoting digestive health and bowel regularity.

Kiwi orange drink can aid in promoting good digestion when coupled with orange juice, which has natural sugars and citric acid that can stimulate digestive enzymes.

Nutrient Density: Fruits like kiwis and oranges are rich in vitamins, minerals, and dietary fiber. You can increase the nutritious content of these fruits and conveniently ingest a range of advantageous components in one glass of juice.

Hydration: Kiwi orange juice, which combines the hydrating properties of orange juice with the water-rich kiwi fruit, can aid in maintaining your hydration. To maintain healthy physical processes and general well-being, it's crucial to stay hydrated.

Cardiovascular Health: Nutrients in oranges and kiwis may help to enhance heart health. Both fruits have low amounts of cholesterol and saturated fat, and their high vitamin C content may help lower the risk of heart disease by supporting normal blood pressure and cholesterol levels.

Lutein and zeaxanthin, two antioxidants known to improve eye health, are abundant in kiwi fruit.

Together with vitamin C and other nutrients found in oranges, these antioxidants can help prevent age-related macular degeneration and advance general eye health.

While kiwi orange juice may provide these possible advantages, it's also critical to have a diversified and balanced diet to make sure you obtain a variety of nutrients from various dietary sources. If you're thinking about buying juice from the store, be aware of portion sizes and additional sugars as well because they can include extra sugars or preservatives.

Recipe
An easy recipe for kiwi orange juice is provided below:

Ingredients:

4 mature kiwis
Oranges, four, huge

Instructions:

1. Prepare the kiwis first. After removing the skin, chop them into small pieces.
2. The oranges should next be squeezed to release their juice. You can squeeze citrus fruits by hand or with a juicer.
3. Fill a blender or food processor with the orange juice that has just been freshly squeezed.
4. Blend the orange juice and kiwi chunks in a blender.
5. High-speed blending is required to properly purée the kiwi and combine it with the orange juice. This process ought to take a minute.
6. Pour the mixture through a fine-mesh filter to get rid of any pulp or seeds once it has been well-blended and smooth. Depending on your preferences, this step is optional.
7. Insert a pitcher or individual serving glasses with the freshly strained kiwi orange juice.
8. The juice can be served immediately over ice or chilled in the refrigerator for a few hours before serving.

You can add a slice of orange or kiwi to the glasses as a garnish if you like.

savor the cooling kiwi orange juice!

Coconut Juice Cabana

Benefits

The clear liquid within young, green coconuts is called coconut cabana juice or coconut water. Due to its reviving flavor and conceivable health advantages, it is a popular beverage in tropical areas and has grown in appeal over the globe. The following are a few advantages of drinking coconut cabana juice:

Hydration: Coconut cabana juice is an all-natural, isotonic beverage with a balance of electrolytes akin to that of human blood. It contains vital electrolytes that support fluid replacement and adequate hydration levels in the body, including potassium, sodium, magnesium, and calcium. It is frequently employed as a natural rehydration remedy to replace fluids lost during physical activity or illness.

Coconut cabana juice is a nutritious substitute for sugary drinks because it is low in calories, fat, and cholesterol. It has important vitamins and minerals like manganese, iron, and zinc, as well as critical elements like vitamins C and B vitamins. It provides a high amount of nutritional fiber as well.

Electrolyte Balance: Potassium and sodium, two electrolytes found in coconut cabana juice, are essential for maintaining healthy fluid balance, neuron function, and muscle contractions. Consuming coconut cabana juice frequently can help the body regain electrolyte equilibrium.

Coconut juice includes antioxidants, like vitamin C, which can assist the body in scavenging dangerous free radicals. Antioxidants assist in decreasing oxidative stress and may improve general health and well-being.

Digestive Health: Coconut coconut juice has a moderate laxative effect and can aid in promoting a healthy digestive system. It contains organic enzymes that facilitate nutrition absorption and digestion. Additionally, normal bowel motions and constipation can be supported by the high fiber content of coconut cabana juice.

Blood Pressure Control: Coconut cabana juice has a higher potassium level than most fruits, which makes it a healthy beverage for people with high blood pressure. Potassium may assist maintain healthy blood pressure levels by balancing the effects of sodium on the body.

Kidney Stone Prevention: According to certain research, drinking coconut cabana juice regularly may help avoid the development of kidney stones. It is thought that naturally occurring components in coconut cabana juice, like potassium citrate, may prevent calcium oxalate, a frequent kidney stone type, from crystallizing.

While coconut cabana juice may have certain advantages, it should not be used as a substitute for a healthy diet and active lifestyle because individual outcomes may differ. Always seek expert medical assistance from a healthcare provider if you have certain health issues or ailments to receive tailored guidance.

Recipe

The following is a recipe for cool Coconut Cabana juice:

Ingredients:

one young coconut
Pineapple juice, 1 cup
half a cup of orange juice
a teaspoon of lime juice
1 tablespoon of optionally sweetening honey or
sugar

Instructions:

1. Open the fresh coconut first. To achieve this,
    sever the coconut's eyes with a knife or
    screwdriver and pour the coconut water into a
    basin. Invest in some coconut water to use
    later.
2. Once the coconut water has been removed,
    carefully crack open the coconut to release
    the flesh. The coconut flesh should be finely
    chopped using a knife or a coconut grater.
    Place aside.
3. Shredded coconut meat, pineapple, orange,
    lime, and sweetener (if using) should all be
    blended. You can drain the coconut milk
    before putting it in the blender for a smoother
    texture.

4. Blend the mixture until it's well-combined and smooth.
5. You can thin out the consistency if it is too thick to your taste by adding more pineapple juice or coconut water.
6. Pour the blended Coconut Cabana juice into glasses once it has reached the appropriate consistency.
7. You can serve the juice plain or top it with a wedge of pineapple or some shredded coconut.

The handmade Coconut Cabana juice is delicious! It is a tropical beverage that is cooling and ideal for hot days.

Apple-Jicama Juice

Benefits

Jicama pear juice is a tasty and healthy drink that has several health advantages. The following are some possible advantages of drinking jicama pear juice:

Jicama pear juice is a wonderful source of vitamins and minerals that are needed for optimum health. Jicama contains a lot of vitamin C, a nutrient essential for collagen formation, immune system health, and antioxidant activity. Vitamins including vitamin K, vitamin C, and potassium, which are necessary for strong bones, a healthy immune system, and a strong heart, can be found in pears.

Jicama pear juice is a hydrating beverage since both jicama and pears are high in water content. To support many biological functions and maintain general health, it's crucial to stay properly hydrated.

Pears and jicama are both fantastic sources of nutritional fiber. Constipation is avoided by fiber, which also aids in healthy digestion. Fiber may also help control blood sugar levels and maintain a healthy weight. Juice made from jicama and pears can help you get the recommended daily allowance of fiber.

Jicama and pears both have antioxidant properties that help the body fend against oxidative stress and lower the risk of chronic illnesses. Free radicals can damage cells, cause inflammation, and contribute to the onset of illness. Antioxidants counteract these dangerous free radicals.

Weight management: Jicama pear juice's low-calorie content and high fiber content can help people feel full longer and help them manage their weight. The high water content can also keep you hydrated and possibly lessen your cravings for calorie-dense beverages.

Juice made from jicama and pears has been shown to support a healthy digestive system. By feeding healthy gut bacteria, the fiber content helps assist regular bowel motions and enhance gut health.

Jicama pear juice should be consumed as part of a healthy diet and lifestyle, even though it may have some potential health benefits. Before making large dietary changes if you have any particular health issues or medical problems, it is always a good idea to speak with a healthcare provider or qualified dietitian.

Recipe

An easy recipe for Jicama Pear Juice is provided below:

Ingredients:

1 jicama, size medium
2 pears
1 lemon
1 to 2 cups of water, as necessary
Ice cubes, if desired
Sweetener, if desired (optional)

Instructions:

1. Jicama should be peeled using a vegetable peeler before being sliced into smaller pieces for your juicer. Place aside.
2. Pears should be cored and divided into smaller pieces.
3. To get the lemon juice, cut the lemon in half and squeeze it. Place aside.
4. Juice the jicama pieces and pears together in a juicer. You can use a blender and later strain the mixture if you don't have a juicer.
5. Add the freshly squeezed lemon juice to the mixture after juicing the jicama and pears.

6. Sweeteners, such as honey or agave syrup, can be added if desired. Start with a little and then increase or decrease as desired.
7. To fully melt the tastes, thoroughly stir the mixture.
8. If the juice seems too thick, gradually add water until the required consistency is reached. Ice cubes can be added to the drink to make it more cooling.
9. Pour the jicama pear juice into glasses and serve immediately after everything has been thoroughly blended.

Juice made with jicama and pears is delicious!

Blackberry Banana Juice

Benefits

Banana blackberry juice has several potential advantages because it combines two healthy fruits. The following are some potential benefits of drinking banana blackberry juice:

Bananas and blackberries are both nutrient-rich foods that are loaded with important vitamins, minerals, and antioxidants. Blackberries are high in vitamin C, vitamin K, manganese, and antioxidants such as anthocyanins, whereas bananas are a good source of vitamin C, potassium, vitamin B6, and dietary fiber.

Antioxidant qualities: Anthocyanins, vitamin C, and other flavonoids, which are antioxidants found in bananas and blackberries, can aid the body fight oxidative stress. Oxidative stress is connected to aging and several chronic diseases. Regular consumption of antioxidants may aid in preventing free radical damage to cells.

Heart health: Bananas' potassium concentration is good for the heart since it helps control blood pressure. Anthocyanins, which are found in blackberries, are linked to a lower risk of heart disease. These fruits may support a healthy cardiovascular system when consumed together.

The health of the digestive system: Bananas and blackberries are both high in dietary fiber. Fiber helps a healthy gut while also assisting in digestion and encouraging regular bowel motions. Juice made from bananas and blackberries can support good digestive health.

Bananas are renowned for their high water content and natural electrolytes like potassium, which support the body's correct electrolyte balance and hydration. Blackberries can provide even more hydration benefits to the drink.

Support for the immune system: Bananas and blackberries both contain vitamin C. It is essential for boosting the immune system and assisting the body in warding off illnesses and infections. Drinking banana blackberry juice frequently may improve your immune system.

Weight loss: Banana blackberry juice, which has little calories, can be a better option than sugary drinks. The fiber content may support weight management attempts by promoting satiety and regulating hunger.

To fully enjoy the advantages of a healthy lifestyle, keep in mind that individual outcomes may vary and that it's always a good idea to eat a diversified diet that contains a range of fruits, vegetables, and other nutritious foods. Additionally, it's wise to speak with a healthcare practitioner for specialized guidance if you have any particular health issues or diseases.

Recipe
An easy recipe for banana blackberry juice is provided below:

Ingredients:

two ripe bananas
Blackberries, 1 cup
one water cup
(Optional and according to taste)
Ice cubes, if desired

Instructions:

1. Peeling bananas is required and cut into pieces.
2. Remove any stems or leaves and rinse the blackberries in cool water.
3. Blend the blackberries and banana bits in a food processor.
4. To the blender, add the water.

5. If you want to sweeten the juice, you can add honey or sugar. Start with a little and then increase or decrease as desired.

6. Blend the ingredients at a high speed until they are well combined and smooth. You can add a bit of extra water if the consistency is too thick.

7. To get rid of any pulp or seeds, you can pass the juice through a fine-mesh sieve if you choose. Since some individuals like pulpier juice, this step is optional.

8. Pour the juice into the glasses and serve right away. For a cooling drink, you can also add some ice cubes.

9. Your homemade banana blackberry juice is delicious!

Chapter 5. Juice Made From Vegetables

I'd be pleased to offer an overview of juices made from vegetables. Given that they are a great source of vitamins, minerals, and antioxidants, vegetable juices are a favorite among those who are concerned about their health. Let's dissect the review into numerous categories:

Juices made from vegetables can have a variety of tastes, depending on the ingredients. While some individuals prefer slightly salty and earthy flavors, others can find them less appetizing than fruit drinks. To improve the flavor and appeal to a wider audience, many brands and recipes combine veggies with fruits or add natural sweeteners.

Nutritional Value: The high nutritional value of juices made from vegetables is one of their main benefits. They are abundant in vitamins A and C, potassium, folate, and dietary fiber, among other important nutrients. A wide range of health advantages from mixing different vegetables can be provided, boosting general well-being.

Juices made from vegetables are said to have several health advantages. The plethora of vitamins and antioxidants can promote heart health while also boosting the immune system, skin health, and digestion. Additionally, the high fiber content may improve intestinal health and help control blood sugar levels.

Freshness and Quality: The freshness and origin of the components have a significant impact on the quality of vegetable juices. Juices that are freshly produced and cold-pressed retain more nutrients than juices that have been pasteurized and industrially processed. Some companies include organic vegetables, which can be a key consideration for consumers who are concerned about their health.

Sugar Content: Although vegetable juices typically contain less sugar than fruit juices, some recipes or commercially available brands may still include fruit juices or other sweeteners for improved flavor. If you want to make sure you're not ingesting too much sugar, it's critical to read the nutrition label and ingredient list.

Dietary Considerations: Most diets, including vegan, vegetarian, and gluten-free ones, can tolerate juices made from vegetables. To be sure there are no potential allergens, anyone with certain dietary restrictions or allergies should carefully review the components.

Due to the expense of materials and processing, fresh vegetable-based juices may be more expensive than other beverages. The cost of store-bought alternatives might vary, with some quality products fetching higher costs.

How much you love vegetable-based juices depends on your unique preferences, just like with any other food or drink. Certain pairings may appeal to some people more than others.

Overall, vegetable-based juices can add value to a balanced diet by making it simple to receive a range of crucial nutrients into your system. Pay attention to the components and the nutritional value of the products, whether you decide to manufacture them at home or purchase them from respected brands. As with any food or beverage, moderation is essential to reap the benefits while keeping in mind your overall nutritional consumption.

These vegetable-based juices can help you healthily lose weight.

Juice From Carrots

Benefits

Due to its high vitamin content, carrot juice is a healthy beverage that provides several health advantages. The following are a few of the main advantages of drinking carrot juice:

Full of nutrients: Beta-carotene, potassium, vitamin C, and vitamin K1 are all found in abundance in carrots, which are also a great source of other critical vitamins and minerals. These nutrients are essential for maintaining several body activities.

Better vision: Due to their high beta-carotene content, carrots are renowned for improving eye health. The body transforms beta-carotene into vitamin A, which is necessary for maintaining good vision, particularly in low-light situations.

Carrot juice has antioxidant effects since it contains beta-carotene, lutein, and zeaxanthin. These substances aid in the body's defense against dangerous free radicals, lowering oxidative stress and maybe reducing the risk of chronic diseases.

Immune system booster: The vitamins and antioxidants in carrot juice can fortify the immune system, assisting the body in more successfully fending off infections and illnesses.

Skin health: Carrot juice's vitamins and antioxidants can help maintain healthy skin by shielding it from UV radiation and other environmental aggressors. They might also make the skin appear more vibrant.

Cardiovascular health: Regularly drinking carrot juice may help to lower blood pressure and cholesterol levels, hence promoting heart health.

Digestive health: Dietary fiber included in carrots helps with digestion and supports a healthy digestive tract. Carrot juice can be helpful for people who have constipation or other digestive problems.

Weight management: Carrot juice has a low-calorie count and might be a useful complement to a diet or exercise regimen.

Carrots include several chemicals that have anti-inflammatory qualities, which may help lessen inflammation in the body and relieve symptoms brought on by inflammatory disorders.

Carrot juice can help you stay properly hydrated by adding to your usual fluid consumption.

While carrot juice has many health advantages, it should be drunk as part of a balanced diet with a variety of foods. It's advisable to speak with a healthcare provider before making any dietary changes or using supplements, especially if you have any underlying medical illnesses or concerns. Moderation is also important since, due to the high beta-carotene concentration, drinking carrot juice may result in "carotenemia," an orange skin coloring.

Recipe

A delicious and healthy beverage that is simple to create at home is carrot juice. Here is a quick recipe for carrot juice:

Ingredients:

4-5 big carrots, preferably organic
1 to 2 cups of water, depending on the desired consistency
Add 1-2 teaspoons of honey or maple syrup, at your discretion, for extra sweetness.
Optional: Add a squeeze of lemon or a piece of ginger for flavor.

Instructions:

1. The carrots should be properly washed in cold running water and peeled if preferred. Since organic carrots typically don't contain dangerous pesticides, you can eat them skin-on.
2. To make the carrots easy to combine, cut them into smaller pieces.
3. Blend the water and the chopped carrots in a blender. You may not require as much water if your blender is powerful. Start with a lower quantity and increase it as necessary to get the required uniformity.
4. Optional step: Pour in the honey or maple syrup for sweetness, and add a little lemon

juice for tang if you'd like. Add a tiny piece of peeled ginger for an added flavor boost.

5. The mixture should be blended at a high speed until the carrots are pureed and the juice is smooth.

6. You can now taste the juice and, if necessary, add more honey, maple syrup, or lemon juice to change its sweetness or sourness.

7. To get a smoother texture, strain the juice through a cheesecloth or fine mesh strainer to get rid of any pulp that is still present. Since many individuals love the juice's fiber content, this step is not required.

8. The carrot juice should be served right away, preferably chilled. If you like it cooler, you may also add ice cubes.

9. Although fresh carrot juice is preferred, any leftovers can be kept for up to 24 hours in the refrigerator. Before consuming, don't forget to shake or stir the juice because natural separation could happen.

Enjoy your homemade carrot juice, a tasty and nutritious way to receive the vitamins and minerals your body needs!

Powerful Sweet Potato Juice

Benefits

A delicious and nutritious addition to your diet can be sweet potato power juice. The following are some possible advantages of drinking sweet potato power juice:

Rich in Nutrients: Sweet potatoes are a great source of potassium, vitamin C, dietary fiber, and vitamin A (in the form of beta-carotene). These nutrients are crucial for supporting various biological processes and preserving overall health.

Sweet potatoes are high in antioxidants like beta-carotene, which assist the body in scavenging dangerous free radicals. Antioxidants can lessen the risk of chronic diseases and shield cells from oxidative stress.

Supports Eye Health: The body converts sweet potatoes' high levels of beta-carotene, which is necessary for healthy vision, into vitamin A. Consuming enough vitamin A helps lower the risk of age-related macular degeneration and maintain eye health.

Boosts Immunity: The combination of vitamins A and C in sweet potatoes enhances the body's resistance to diseases and infections by boosting the immune system.

Sweet potatoes are an excellent source of dietary fiber, which supports a healthy digestive system and regular bowel motions. Additionally, fiber can lower blood sugar and lessen post-meal increases.

Supports Heart Health: Potassium, which is present in sweet potatoes, supports heart health by regulating blood pressure and lowering the risk of heart attack and stroke.

Increased Energy: Sweet potatoes are an excellent source of complex carbs that release energy gradually throughout the day. Because of this, sweet potato power juice is a fantastic choice for athletes and those who lead active lives.

Antioxidants and vitamins found in sweet potatoes help to maintain healthy, glowing skin. They assist in preventing skin aging, enhancing skin texture, and preserving a radiant complexion.

Anti-Inflammatory qualities: Some sweet potato chemicals, like anthocyanins, have anti-inflammatory qualities that may be useful in lowering inflammatory responses in the body.

You can increase the nutritional content of sweet potato power juice by including other nutritious ingredients like ginger, turmeric, or a dash of citrus juice. It's crucial to remember that juice shouldn't completely replace whole sweet potatoes in your diet because the fiber value is diminished. Instead, think about including sweet potato power juice into a healthy diet to benefit from any potential health advantages. A healthcare expert should be consulted before making any dietary changes, especially if you have any particular health conditions or worries.

Recipe

Here is a recipe for a tasty and nutritious sweet potato power drink:

Ingredients:

Peeled and diced one medium-sized sweet potato
2 big, peeled, and chopped carrots
1 cored and cut red apple
Peeled, fresh ginger, 1 inch long
Peeled and seeded lemon, 1
1 cup of water or coconut water, adjusted for
consistency, as needed

Optional additions for more flavor and nutrition:

Unseed and peel 1 small orange.
a dash of turmeric or cinnamon
Adding a little cayenne pepper for some heat

Instructions:

1. As directed in the list above, wash and
   prepare each ingredient.
2. Feed the sweet potato, carrots, apple, ginger,
   and lemon (and optional orange if using)
   through the juicer one at a time using a
   high-quality juicer.
3. Put the juice in a pitcher or container.

4. Add coconut water or water if you prefer a thinner consistency, and stir well. You can change the amount to suit your tastes.
5. Stir any optional ingredients you choose to use into the juice for flavor and health benefits.
6. The sweet potato power juice is ready to drink once it has been poured into glasses.
7. Don't forget to drink the juice right away for maximum nutritional impact. Add some ice cubes or place the juice in the refrigerator for a short period before serving if you prefer your juice cooler. Take pleasure in your delicious and nourishing sweet potato power juice!

Beet Juice With Ginger

Benefits

A healthy beverage called ginger beet juice is created by blending or juicing fresh ginger and beets. Beets and ginger each have several health advantages, and when blended into a beverage, those advantages can increase. The following are some potential advantages of ginger beet juice:

Beets and ginger are both nutrient-rich foods that are loaded with important vitamins, minerals, and antioxidants. While ginger includes vitamin C, magnesium, and potassium, beets are a wonderful source of folate, manganese, potassium, and vitamin C.

Improved digestion: The digestive advantages of ginger are well established. It can help relieve gastrointestinal irritation, lessen bloating, and ease indigestion. Beets are also rich in fiber, which promotes a healthy digestive system.

Enhanced immune system: The vitamin C and antioxidants in ginger and beets can help your body fight off infections and illnesses by boosting your immune system.

Inflammation reduction: Ginger and beets both contain anti-inflammatory qualities that might aid in reducing inflammation in the body. Including anti-inflammatory items in your diet can be useful because chronic inflammation is connected to several health problems.

Detoxification: The natural detoxification activities of the liver are supported by the chemicals found in beets. Drinking ginger beet juice may help the body remove toxins.

Blood pressure reduction: According to some research, drinking beet juice may help lower blood pressure since it contains a lot of nitrates, which can relax and widen blood vessels.

Improved exercise performance: It has been demonstrated that the nitrates in beets increase blood flow and oxygen supply to muscles, potentially enhancing endurance.

Beets and ginger are both thought to be heart-healthy meals. Beets' nitrate concentration may promote cardiovascular health, and the antioxidants in ginger may lower the risk of heart disease.

Cognitive function: According to some research, ginger's antioxidants may have neuroprotective qualities that are beneficial to brain health and cognitive function.

It's important to remember that while ginger beet juice may have certain health advantages, it should only be used as a part of a healthy, balanced diet. A healthcare practitioner should be consulted before making any dietary changes or using any supplements, especially if you have any pre-existing medical conditions or are taking medication. It's also important to be aware of any possible allergies or sensitivities to these substances because ginger beet juice may not be suited for everyone.

Recipe

Here is a recipe for delicious and healthy ginger beet juice:

Ingredients:

Wash, peel, and cut 2 medium-sized beets.
1 inch of freshly peeled ginger root
two big carrots, cleaned and cut
1 cored and chopped apple
Juiced lemon, one

1 cup of water (or more, depending on the
consistency you want)
Ice cubes, if desired

Instructions:

1. Wash, peel, and chop each ingredient as needed to complete the preparation.
2. The juice from the apple, carrots, ginger, and beets should be extracted using a juicer. In the absence of a juicer, you can also use a powerful blender and strain the juice through a fine mesh strainer or nut milk bag.
3. Combine the freshly extracted juice, lemon juice, and water in a pitcher or other container. Depending on how powerful or diluted you want the juice to be, you can change the amount of water.
4. To ensure that the flavors are dispersed equally, thoroughly stir the mixture.
5. If you'd like the juice to be cool and refreshing, add some ice cubes.
6. To reap the most nutritious benefits, pour the ginger-beet juice into glasses and serve right away.

Note: Use caution when handling beet juice to prevent stains on surfaces and clothing. To maintain the nutrients and flavor, it is essential to consume the juice as soon as it is produced. However, you can keep any juice that is left over for up to 24 hours in the refrigerator. If it separates, give it a vigorous shake before consuming. Enjoy your wholesome, colorful ginger-beet juice!

Tomato Juice With Heat

Benefits

A drink known as spicy tomato juice is created by combining tomato juice with various spices, most often chili peppers or hot sauces. The combination of tomatoes and spices may have the following advantages:

Rich in Nutrients: Lycopene and other antioxidants including vitamins A, C, and K can be found in tomato juice along with other important nutrients.

These nutrients assist immune system function, skin health, and other aspects of general health.

Digestion: The tomato juice's spice might stimulate the digestive tract and aid in better digestion. It might improve gut health and lessen indigestion symptoms.

Weight management: Spicy foods, such as hot tomato juice, might momentarily speed up metabolism and encourage fullness. Through a reduction in total calorie intake, this may aid in weight management.

Lycopene, an antioxidant found in tomatoes, has been related to improvements in heart health. The risk of heart disease may be reduced by lowering blood pressure and lowering levels of harmful cholesterol.

Capsaicin, the primary ingredient in chili peppers that gives them their spiciness, also has anti-inflammatory benefits. This might help treat diseases brought on by inflammation.

Spicy foods can improve circulation by promoting greater blood flow throughout the body.

Pain relief: According to certain research, capsaicin may lessen pain by obstructing specific pain signals in the body.

Support for the Immune System: The vitamins and antioxidants in tomato juice can help boost the immune system, enabling the body to fend against diseases and infections.

Hydration: Tomato juice is a hydrating beverage choice due to its high water content.

Despite these possible advantages, it's important to keep in mind that everyone's reaction to spicy meals will be different. After ingesting spicy tomato juice, some people may develop discomfort, heartburn, or digestive problems. Additionally, people who suffer from illnesses like acid reflux or irritable bowel syndrome (IBS) may not be able to consume spicy tomato juice. To make sure that your dietary changes support your health needs and goals, it is best to speak with a healthcare provider or registered dietitian.

Recipe

Here is a quick recipe for hot tomato juice:

Ingredients:

4 cups chopped, fresh, and ripe tomatoes or tomato
juice
1-2 minced garlic cloves
1 small onion, diced finely
1-2 finely sliced celery stalks
1-2 small carrots, peeled and cut finely
Lemon juice, 1 to 2 teaspoons (adjust to taste)
Worcestershire sauce, one teaspoon
1 teaspoon hot sauce (such as Sriracha or Tabasco);
adjust the amount to your preferred level of heat.
a half-teaspoon of black pepper, ground
Add taste-tested salt, roughly about half a teaspoon.
(This is optional) 1/4 teaspoon cayenne pepper for
more spiciness
For garnish, use fresh herbs like basil or cilantro.
Ice cubes, if desired

Instructions:

1. Wash and chop fresh tomatoes into small pieces if you're using them. You can omit this step if you are using tomato juice.
2. Combine the chopped tomatoes (or tomato juice), minced garlic, diced onion, celery, and carrots in a blender or food processor. Blend the mixture until it's smooth.
3. To separate the pulp from the juice, pour the blended liquid into a sizable pitcher or a fine-mesh strainer set over a basin. To get the most juice out of the mixture, press down on it with a spoon.
4. To the tomato liquid, mix in the lemon juice, Worcestershire sauce, spicy sauce, salt, black pepper, and cayenne pepper (if using). To completely meld the flavors, stir well.
5. as per your preferences, taste the tomato juice and adjust the seasonings. If necessary, add more lemon juice, spicy sauce, or salt.
6. If preferred, chill the juice using ice cubes in the pitcher or chill it for an hour before serving.
7. Give the hot tomato juice a vigorous stir before serving as some settling may take place.

8. Pour the hot tomato juice into glasses and top with fresh cilantro or basil to serve.

9. Savor the spicy tomato juice you produced at home! You can further strain the juice before serving if you like pulp-free juice. Feel free to experiment with various spices and ingredients to make this dish your own.

Cucumber-Celery Juice

Benefits

Juice made from cucumbers and celery combines the moisturizing qualities of cucumbers with the nutrient-dense qualities of celery to create a popular health drink. It's important to remember that there has been little scientific research on the precise advantages of this juice blend, despite promises about its possible health benefits. The following are some potential advantages of drinking cucumber-celery juice:

Cucumbers and celery both contain a lot of water, so juice is a great method to stay hydrated and keep the body's fluid balance in check.

Cucumbers and celery are low in calories but high in nutrients, including potassium, folate, vitamin C, vitamin K, and vitamin. A handy approach to consuming these minerals is by drinking the juice.

Cucumbers and celery both have antioxidant characteristics, including flavonoids, tannins, and vitamin C, which might help the body fight off dangerous free radicals and possibly lessen oxidative stress.

Cucurbitacins and phytosterols, two substances present in cucumbers and celery, have been examined for their possible anti-inflammatory actions, which may help to lessen inflammation in the body.

Digestive health: Due to their high fiber content, cucumbers are a popular food that can help with digestive health by encouraging regular bowel movements and reducing constipation.

Weight management: Cucumber celery juice can be a delightful and filling beverage that may help in weight control attempts by reducing overall calorie intake. This is due to their low calorie and high water content.

Skin health: The vitamin C and silica in cucumber celery juice may be good for the skin, boosting the development of collagen and fostering a radiant complexion.

It's crucial to keep in mind that although these possible advantages appear promising, additional research is required to substantiate the precise health benefits of cucumber celery juice. It should not be used as a substitute for a balanced and varied diet because individual reactions to this juice blend may differ.

It's always a good idea to speak with a healthcare provider or a trained nutritionist if you're thinking about including cucumber celery juice into your daily routine to make sure it complements your health objectives and any existing ailments you might have.

Recipe

A quick and tasty recipe for cucumber celery juice is provided below:

Ingredients:

1-inch cucumber
4-5 stalks of celery
12 a lemon, optionally, for flavor
(Optional) Fresh mint leaves add a sense of freshness
(Optional) Ice cubes for a cold juice

Instructions:

1. Under cold running water, give the cucumber, celery stalks, lemon, and mint leaves a good wash.
2. Trim the ends of the celery stalks and chop the cucumber into bits.
3. Feed the cucumber and celery through the juicer one at a time if you're using one to extract the juice from them. You can use a blender and afterward strain the juice if you don't have a juicer.

4. Cucumber and celery chunks should be added to a blender along with a little bit of water, and the mixture should be blended until smooth. To remove the juice, next strain the mixture through a cheesecloth, fine mesh strainer, or nut milk bag. Extract as much juice as you can.

5. If using, cut the lemon in half and juice each half separately. Depending on how much lemon juice you desire, you can vary the amount.

6. If using mint, tear a few leaves and incorporate them with the cucumber and celery mixture. Although it is optional, this step gives the dish a lovely freshness.

7. In a glass, pour the juice that was extracted. For cold juice, if preferred, add ice cubes.

To get the juice's full nutritional advantages, thoroughly stir it before drinking.
Juice made from cucumber and celery is not only hydrating but also rich in antioxidants, vitamins, and minerals. It's a fantastic choice for a healthful and energizing beverage, especially during the sweltering summer months. Enjoy

Juice Of Red Cabbage With Carrots

Benefits

When ingested as a part of a balanced diet, red cabbage, and carrot juice can provide several health advantages. Both vegetables are abundant in crucial minerals and phytochemicals that support general health. The following are a few potential advantages of red cabbage and carrot juice:

Red cabbage and carrots are both good suppliers of vitamins and minerals, including potassium, manganese, vitamin K, vitamin A, and vitamin C. These nutrients are crucial for supporting bone health, fostering good blood coagulation, preserving healthy skin, and bolstering the immune system.

Both veggies are high in antioxidants including anthocyanins and carotenoids like beta-carotene, lutein, and zeaxanthin. These antioxidants aid in the body's defense against dangerous free radicals, reducing oxidative stress and inflammation while possibly lowering the risk of developing chronic illnesses.

Supports heart health: By regulating blood pressure and enhancing blood vessel function, the potassium in carrot juice and the anthocyanins in red cabbage juice may enhance heart health.

The health of the digestive system: Dietary fiber found in carrot juice can help with digestion and support a healthy gut. Additionally, it might aid in promoting regular bowel motions and preventing constipation.

Eye health: Carrots are well-known for having a high concentration of beta-carotene, which the body transforms into vitamin A. Vitamin A is essential for keeping clear vision and may lower the risk of cataracts and age-related macular degeneration.

Red cabbage and carrots include components that support the body's natural detoxification processes, assisting in the removal of toxins and toxic substances. These substances include glucosinolates and sulfur-containing compounds.

Some research indicates that the antioxidants and other substances present in red cabbage and carrots may have anti-cancer capabilities and may help lower the chance of developing some types of cancer.

Weight management: Red cabbage and carrot juice can be a calorie-efficient approach to increase the number of important nutrients in your diet, which may help with weight management and promote general health.

Red cabbage and carrot juice can both be beneficial for your health, but they should only be consumed as a part of a well-balanced diet that also includes an additional variety of other vegetables, Fruits, complete grains, and lean proteins. Also, keep in mind that certain vegetables may cause allergies or sensitivities in some people. Before making significant dietary changes if you have any particular health issues or diseases, it is always a good idea to speak with a medical practitioner or a qualified dietitian.

Recipe

Red cabbage carrot juice combines the health advantages of both red cabbage and carrots into one tasty, vibrant beverage. Here is the straightforward recipe for this energizing juice:

Ingredients:

50% of a tiny red cabbage
3-inch-long carrots
One apple, optionally, for sweetness
Fresh ginger, cut into 1-inch pieces, optional (for taste).
(As needed) Water

Instructions:

1. To get rid of any dirt or contaminants, thoroughly wash all of the vegetables.
2. To make the red cabbage fit smoothly into your juicer chute, cut it into smaller pieces.
3. The carrots should be peeled and chopped into smaller pieces.
4. Remove the core and seeds from the apple before cutting them into pieces.
5. Ginger should be peeled and chopped into small pieces.

6. Start juicing by adding one ingredient at a time to the juicer: red cabbage, carrots, apple (if used), and ginger (if used).
7. Gather the juice in a glass or a pitcher.
8. If the juice is too concentrated, you can add extra water to dilute it and get the consistency you want.
9. Stir the juice before serving.
10. In glasses, pour the red cabbage and carrot juice.

Please take note that you can modify the amounts of red cabbage, carrots, and other ingredients to suit your personal preferences. If you're not accustomed to the earthy flavor of red cabbage, adding an apple can make the juice sweeter and more delectable.

If you want a milder flavor, you may eliminate the ginger, although it does give some pleasant zing and additional health benefits. To gain the maximum nutritious benefit from the fresh ingredients, it's also preferable to drink the juice right away after making it. If there are any leftovers, you may keep the juice in the fridge for up to 24 hours by sealing it in a jar. Don't forget to thoroughly swirl it before each subsequent drink.

Enjoy this red cabbage and carrot juice's bright hues and health advantages!

Green Ginger Juice

Benefits

Ginger green juice is a wholesome drink that combines the advantages of ginger and green vegetables for your health. Although individual outcomes may differ, the following are some possible advantages of ginger green juice:

Ginger has anti-inflammatory properties because it includes bioactive substances like gingerol. Juice made from ginger may help lower inflammation in the body, which may be helpful for those with inflammatory illnesses and conditions like arthritis.

Ginger has long been used to treat digestive problems like indigestion, bloating, and motion sickness. The juice can offer extra fiber and nutrients that assist good digestion when mixed with green vegetables.

Green vegetables like spinach, kale, and cucumber are abundant in antioxidants, which aid in the body's defense against dangerous free radicals. This might aid in lowering oxidative stress and advancing general health.

Immune System Booster: Excellent sources of vitamins and minerals that support the immune system include both ginger and green vegetables. Ginger green juice regularly may aid to bolster your body's defense mechanisms.

Green vegetables and ginger together may help the body cleanse itself by promoting healthy liver function and assisting in the removal of pollutants.

Weight management: Green vegetables are low in calories and abundant in nutrients, so drinking ginger green juice while trying to control your weight is a good idea.

Improved Hydration: Especially in hot weather or after exercise, drinking ginger green juice can be a refreshing way to stay hydrated.

Cardiovascular Support: According to some studies, ginger consumption as part of a balanced diet may help lower cholesterol levels and increase blood circulation, which may be beneficial for heart health.

It's crucial to remember that while ginger green juice might have several health advantages, a well-balanced diet should always come first. Individual sensitivity to ginger or specific green vegetables may also occur, so it's best to pay attention to how the juice affects your body and get medical advice if you have any worries or a history of illnesses.

Recipe

Here is a quick and tasty recipe for ginger green juice:

Ingredients:

1 small cucumber
fresh spinach greens, 2 cups
2-3 celery stalks
Fresh ginger root, 1 to 2 inches long (adjust to taste)
1 apple green
1 lemon

Instructions:

1. To get rid of any dirt or pollutants, properly wash all the fruits and vegetables.
2. For simpler blending, peel the ginger root and cut it into small pieces.
3. Slice the apple into chunks after coring it.
4. Cucumber and celery should be chopped into smaller bits.
5. Remove any seeds before squeezing the juice from the cut-in-half lemon.
6. Juice or combine the cucumber, spinach, celery, ginger, apple, and lemon juice.
7. The mixture must be smooth and constant before you may drink it.
8. To create a smoother juice if you're using a blender, you might need to strain the liquid through a fine mesh strainer.

9. The ginger green juice can be chilled or
    served right away over ice for a cool and
    nutritious beverage.

To preserve their nutritious worth, fresh juices
should be drunk as soon as possible after
preparation. Enjoy this nutrient-rich ginger green
juice as a tasty addition to your day.

Gazpacho Tomato Juice

Benefits

A common chilly soup made with fresh tomatoes,
cucumbers, bell peppers, onions, garlic, and olive oil
is called tomato gazpacho juice. Usually, salt,
pepper, and vinegar are used to season it. Because of
its nutrient-rich contents, this hydrating and healthy
beverage provides several health advantages. The
following are some potential advantages of tomato
gazpacho juice:

Rich in vitamins and minerals: Tomatoes are a fantastic source of vitamins and minerals, particularly folate, potassium, vitamin C, and vitamin K. These nutrients are crucial for immune system health, blood coagulation, heart health, and general well-being.

Tomatoes are abundant in antioxidants including lycopene, beta-carotene, and vitamin C which assist the body in scavenging dangerous free radicals. Particularly, lycopene has been linked to a lower risk of developing some malignancies and may benefit skin health.

Gazpacho juice contains a substantial amount of water from the fresh vegetables used in its preparation, making it a hydrating beverage. Overall health depends on staying hydrated, and gazpacho can be a delightful method to help you meet your daily water requirements.

Heart Health: The monounsaturated fats and nutrients in gazpacho, which are derived from the mixture of tomatoes and olive oil, may lower LDL cholesterol levels and lower the chance of developing heart disease.

Weight management: Gazpacho often has a low-calorie count and a high fiber content, which can aid in satiety and improve weight loss attempts. The presence of fiber facilitates digestion and increases how long you feel full.

Improved Digestion: The vegetables in gazpacho, particularly bell peppers, and cucumbers, are abundant in water and fiber, which helps assist good digestion.

Reduced Inflammation: The anti-inflammatory characteristics of several ingredients in gazpacho, like tomatoes and garlic, may help lessen chronic inflammation in the body.

Skin Health: By shielding the skin from oxidative stress and promoting collagen formation, tomatoes' antioxidant content and vitamin C can help to improve skin health.

Nutritional Absorption: The good fats in gazpacho, which are derived from olive oil, can help the body absorb fat-soluble vitamins (such as vitamins A and E) from the vegetables used to make the soup.

While tomato gazpacho juice has several health advantages, it should not be used as a substitute for a nutritious diet and active lifestyle. It's usually important to read the ingredient list and use homemade versions whenever feasible because certain store-bought gazpacho juices could have additional sweeteners or high levels of sodium.

Recipe

A cool soup that is both hydrating and nourishing, tomato gazpacho juice is ideal for hot summer days. Here is a quick and delectable meal you should try:

Ingredients:

6 large, chopped, ripe tomatoes
1 chopped and peeled cucumber
1 chopped red bell pepper
1 minced tiny red onion
2 to 3 minced garlic cloves
3 cups tomato juice or homemade or store-bought vegetable broth

Extra virgin olive oil, 1/4 cup
Red wine vinegar, 2 teaspoons (adjust to taste)
1 teaspoon of sugar, optionally used to counteract the acidity
To taste, add salt and black pepper.
garnishing with fresh herbs like basil, parsley, or cilantro

Instructions:

1. Wash and finely cut the tomatoes, cucumbers, red bell peppers, and red onions as you prepare the other vegetables. The garlic cloves are minced.
2. Add the minced garlic and the chopped veggies to a blender or food processor.
3. Vegetables should be blended until smooth or with the appropriate consistency. Blend it less, leaving some small chunks if you prefer a chunkier texture.
4. Olive oil, red wine vinegar, and tomato juice or vegetable broth should all be added to the blender. To keep the gazpacho chilly, use refrigerated tomato juice if using it.
5. You can add a teaspoon of sugar to the gazpacho to balance the flavors if you find it

to be a little too sour or acidic to your taste. If necessary, add more salt and black pepper to the dish's flavoring.

6. To completely integrate all the components, blend the mixture just once more.

7. If required, taste the gazpacho and adjust the seasoning. To fit your flavor preferences, you can increase the amount of salt, vinegar, or olive oil.

8. Transfer the gazpacho fluid to a big pitcher or container once you're happy with the flavor.

9. Before serving, chill the gazpacho in the fridge for at least two to three hours to let the flavors mingle and the soup gets nice and cold.

10. Give the gazpacho a thorough swirl before serving, then ladle it into individual bowls or glasses.

11. Add fresh herbs like basil, parsley, or cilantro as a garnish to the gazpacho for a touch of color and freshness.

12. Take pleasure in your homemade tomato gazpacho as a tasty appetizer or a cool beverage on a hot day. It's ideal for serving at summertime gatherings like barbecues and picnics.

Avocado Spirulina Juice

Benefits

Due to the special qualities and nutrients included in each ingredient, combining spirulina and avocado in a juice can provide several health advantages. The following are some possible advantages of spirulina avocado juice:

Spirulina, a type of blue-green algae, is incredibly rich in nutrients, including protein, vitamins (including vitamin K and B vitamins), minerals (such as iron, magnesium, and potassium), and antioxidants. Avocados are also a great source of nutrients, especially fiber, potassium, healthy monounsaturated fats, and vitamins C, E, K, and B-6.

Phycocyanin, which is found in spirulina, has been demonstrated to have immune-boosting characteristics. This drink can nourish and fortify the immune system by combining avocado's antioxidants and vitamin C.

Spirulina has been investigated for its ability to assist in detoxification by assisting the body in removing heavy metals and other pollutants. Glutathione, a potent antioxidant found in avocado, aids in the detoxification process.

Spirulina is a strong source of iron and plant-based protein, which can help boost one's energy and stamina. Healthy fats included in avocados aid in long-lasting energy and satiety.

Heart Health: Because they help to reduce levels of harmful cholesterol, avocados' monounsaturated fats have been linked to improved heart health. Spirulina may benefit cardiovascular health by lowering blood pressure and enhancing lipid profiles.

Anti-Inflammatory Components: Spirulina and avocado both include anti-inflammatory elements that may help lessen bodily inflammation and treat associated diseases.

Constipation prevention and support: Avocados are a good source of dietary fiber, which promotes healthy digestive health. In addition, spirulina has digestive enzymes in it.

Weight control: By reducing hunger cravings, **the** protein, healthy fats, and fiber in spirulina avocado juice can assist to increase satiety and aid in weight management.

For maximum flavor and nutritional value, spirulina avocado juice must be made with ripe avocados and high-quality, food-grade spirulina powder. Even though this juice can be a nourishing addition to your diet, it's crucial to keep in mind that it shouldn't be used as a substitute for a balanced and diverse diet.

Before making any dietary changes, as with the use of any dietary supplement or novel food, it is wise to speak with a medical expert or qualified dietitian, particularly if you have any existing medical ailments or concerns.

Recipe

Here is a recipe for cool Spirulina Avocado Juice:

Ingredients:

1 mature avocado
fresh spinach leaves, 1 cup
one ripe banana
1/fourth cup of spirulina powder
1 cup of the milk of your choice, such as almond
milk
1 tablespoon of honey or maple syrup, sweetened if
desired
Ice cubes, if desired

Instructions:

1. Cut the avocado in half, remove the pit, and
    then scoop the flesh into a blender.
2. Fresh spinach leaves should be added to the
    blender.
3. The banana should be peeled and added to
    the blender as well.
4. Add the milk of your choice, including
    almond milk.
5. Spirulina powder should be added to the
    blender. Spirulina is a nutrient-dense

superfood, but because of its strong flavor, you should modify the amount to suit your tastes.

6. You can add honey or maple syrup to the mixture for a sweeter flavor.
7. Until the mixture is creamy and smooth, blend all the components. To achieve the required texture, add extra milk if the mixture is too thick.
8. Add a few ice cubes to the blender if you want your juice cold, then blitz again until the ice is crushed and well combined.
9. Pour the Spirulina Avocado Juice into glasses after it has been blended to your preferences and serve right away.

This juice is a terrific choice for a healthy and invigorating beverage because it is not only delectable but also loaded with nutrients from spinach, avocado, and spirulina. Enjoy!

Red Bell Pepper Juice with Carrots

Benefits

Due to their nutritious content, red bell pepper and carrot juice can provide several health advantages. Let's look at some possible advantages of ingesting this juice:

Vitamin-rich: Carrots and red bell peppers are both rich in important vitamins. Red bell peppers are a great source of vitamin C, which helps to build collagen, boost the immune system, and protect the body from oxidative stress. Beta-carotene, a precursor to vitamin A that is necessary for good vision, immune system function, and skin, is abundant in carrots.

Strong antioxidant capabilities are provided by the combination of beta-carotene from carrots and vitamin C from red bell peppers. Antioxidants assist the body in scavenging dangerous free radicals, minimizing cellular damage, and lowering the risk of chronic illnesses.

Eye Health: Because of its high beta-carotene concentration, carrots are frequently linked to better eye health. The body transforms beta-carotene into vitamin A, which is essential for keeping excellent vision, particularly in low-light situations.

Skin Health: Red bell peppers' vitamin C aids in the manufacture of collagen, a protein necessary for preserving skin suppleness and general skin health. Additionally, carrots' beta-carotene may help safeguard skin against sun damage and support a healthy complexion.

Heart Health: By lowering oxidative stress and inflammation, the antioxidants in red bell peppers and carrots help improve heart health. Furthermore, carrots' fiber content may assist control cholesterol levels, enhancing cardiovascular health.

Support for the Immune System: Red bell peppers' vitamin C concentration can boost the body's defenses against infections and disease.

Red bell peppers and carrots both have a high water content, which aids in hydrating the body and aids in digestion. Additionally, the fiber in them promotes a healthy gut and helps with digestion.

Weight management: Red bell pepper and carrot juice have a low-calorie count and can be a useful supplement to a weight loss program because it delivers necessary nutrients without adding unnecessary calories.

Use only fresh, premium products for producing red bell pepper and carrot juice. The juice can be consumed alone or combined with other fruits and vegetables to produce various flavor profiles. It's advisable to speak with a healthcare provider before making any dietary changes, especially if you have any particular health issues or diseases.

Recipe

Recipe for Red Bell Pepper and Carrot Juice:

Ingredients:

two substantial red peppers
4 big carrots
One inch of fresh ginger, optionally, for flavor
Ice cubes, if desired

Instructions:

1. Under running water, give the carrots and red bell peppers a thorough washing. Cut the bell peppers into bits after removing the seeds and stems. For simpler juicing, peel the carrots and chop them into smaller pieces.
2. Peel and cut ginger into smaller chunks if you're using it.
3. Install your juicer as directed by the manufacturer.
4. Red bell peppers should be juiced first, then carrots, and finally ginger (if used). The ingredients will be processed in this order to get the most juice possible while avoiding any obstructions.
5. Give the mixture a vigorous toss to uniformly distribute the flavors after all the ingredients have been juiced.
6. Add ice cubes to the drink and mix once more if you prefer your juice chilly.
7. Red bell pepper and carrot juice should be poured into glasses and served right away. Juice that has just been prepared is always best because it has more nutrients.
8. Graze on your colorful and nourishing red bell pepper and carrot juice! It is a good

source of minerals, vitamins, and antioxidants that are good for your health.

Lime-Spinach Juice

Benefits

Due to the combination of these healthy elements, spinach lime juice can provide several health advantages. Here are a few possible advantages:

Rich in vitamins and minerals: Spinach is a great source of minerals like iron, calcium, and magnesium as well as critical vitamins like vitamins A, C, and K. Lime is a great source of vitamin C as well. This juice can support strong bones, improve skin health, and strengthen your immune system.

Antioxidant qualities: Both spinach and lime include antioxidants that aid in the body's defense against dangerous free radicals, lowering oxidative stress and potential cell damage. Antioxidants are well known for lowering the risk of chronic diseases and enhancing general health.

Hydration: A tasty and hydrating beverage made of lime juice and spinach is beneficial for maintaining normal bodily processes and good health.

Enhances digestion: Citric acid, which is present in lime juice, helps digestion by encouraging the release of digestive fluids. Due to its high fiber content, spinach can help maintain a healthy digestive system and bowel movements.

Spinach's low-calorie count and fiber content might help you feel full and satisfied, supporting weight management. Lime juice may be a valuable addition to a weight loss strategy because it can flavor the beverage without adding extra calories.

Heart health: Potassium and folate, two nutrients found in spinach and lime, can help maintain heart health by controlling blood pressure and lowering the risk of cardiovascular diseases.

Due to its alkaline nature, lime juice can assist maintain the pH balance of the body. Alkaline-rich diets may be good for the bones and may help prevent several chronic diseases.

Although spinach lime juice can be a beneficial addition to your diet, it is still important to have a balanced, diversified diet to obtain a variety of nutrients. Before making big changes to your diet, it's also a good idea to speak with a healthcare provider or a qualified dietitian if you have any particular health conditions or worries.

Recipe

With the benefits of spinach and the tart taste of lime, spinach lime juice is a revitalizing and wholesome beverage. Here is a straightforward recipe for this delicious beverage:

Ingredients:

2 cups of clean, stemmed fresh spinach leaves
Depending on your taste, 2 to 3 limes
two cups of iced water
1-2 teaspoons of honey or any other preferred sweetener
Ice cubes, if desired

Instructions:

1. To prepare the spinach, properly rinse it under cold water to get rid of any dirt or contaminants. The juice may become bitter if the stems are left in.
2. Lime juice can be extracted by hand or with a juicer after the limes have been cut in half. You can squeeze the limes with your hands or a citrus reamer. Eliminate any seeds that may float to the juice's surface.
3. Blend spinach and water: Place the spinach leaves and the water in a blender. Blend the spinach and water at high speed until the spinach is pureed.
4. The combination should be strained through a fine mesh strainer or a nut milk bag if you want smoother juice. To get the most liquid out of the solids, apply pressure.
5. Add the freshly squeezed lime juice to the strained spinach mixture to combine the lime juice. To blend, thoroughly stir.
6. Add honey or any other sweetener of your choosing if you find the juice to be too tart. To suit your preferences, adjust the sweetness.
7. Transfer the spinach lime juice to a pitcher, chill for at least 30 minutes, and then serve. If

you want to serve it right away, you can also add ice cubes.

8. Enjoy: Pour the cooled spinach lime juice into glasses, add a lime slice as a garnish if you like, and sip on your wholesome and revitalizing green beverage!

The lime offers a citrus flavor to counter the earthiness of the greens while the spinach provides a wealth of vitamins, minerals, and antioxidants. It's a fantastic method to increase your intake of greens and give yourself an energy boost.

Protein Energy Drink

Benefits

Protein power juice, sometimes referred to as protein shakes or protein smoothies, is a type of beverage that blends a variety of fruits, vegetables, and other nutritional elements with protein powder to provide a concentrated supply of the amino acid. Athletes, fitness fanatics, and others trying to augment their protein consumption have all grown fond of these drinks. The following are some possible advantages of ingesting protein power juice:

Protein is crucial for the repair and development of muscles following physical exertion. Protein power juice, especially when taken after a workout, can assist in promoting muscle growth and recuperation, which is important for athletes and those who regularly exercise.

Satiety: Protein is believed to increase satiety more so than fats or carbohydrates. You can feel filled for longer by drinking protein-power juice as a snack or meal replacement, which lowers your risk of overeating and supports weight management or weight loss efforts.

Nutrition that is convenient and quick:
Protein-power juice can be a quick and easy method to get a substantial quantity of protein and other nutrients in a single serving. It's especially helpful for people who lead hectic lives or in situations where there aren't many whole-food options.

Protein power juice can be a nutrient-rich beverage, offering vitamins, minerals, and antioxidants necessary for general health and well-being when made with fruits, vegetables, and other beneficial components.

Supports active lifestyles: Protein power juice can be an effective way for people who engage in physical activities like athletics, weightlifting, or endurance training to replace the nutrients and energy they lose while exercising.

Enhanced muscle protein synthesis: Consuming protein power juice can promote muscle protein synthesis, which strengthens and repairs muscle fibers, improving athletic performance and other functional capacities.

Blood sugar control: The protein and carbohydrates in protein power juice work together to stabilize blood sugar levels, making it a possible good choice for people with diabetes or those trying to control their blood sugar levels.

However, it's crucial to keep the following things in mind:

Protein power juice can be helpful, but it shouldn't be the only source of nutrients. The keywords here are balance and moderation. For optimal health, a balanced diet made up of a variety of nutritious foods is necessary.

Consider the protein powder and other items you use in your protein power juice for quality. Select high-quality protein sources and stay away from artificial additives and extra sugar.

Individual needs: The amount of protein needed varies by age, sex, level of activity, and general health. To determine the proper protein consumption for your unique needs, it is recommended to speak with a medical practitioner or a qualified dietitian.

Certain protein sources and other commonly found additives in protein-power juice may cause allergies or sensitivities in some people. Always be conscious of any food intolerances or allergies you may have and modify the recipe as necessary.

In conclusion, protein-power juice can be a helpful supplement to your diet, particularly when utilized as a part of a healthy, wholesome eating regimen that supports your fitness and health goals. Making informed decisions and taking into account your unique demands is crucial when making any dietary changes or supplementation.

Recipe

Here is a recipe for a protein-rich juice that mixes a variety of ingredients to make a nice and healthy drink:

Ingredients:
1 cup of almonds without sugar, milk (or your preferred plant-based milk)
one ripe banana
Greek yogurt, or a dairy-free substitute, in 1/2 cup
Oats, rolled, 14 cup
1 tablespoon natural almond or peanut butter
Chia seeds, one tablespoon
maple syrup, 1 tbsp or honey (optional, for extra sweetness)
One-half teaspoon of vanilla extract
(Optional) Ice cubes for a chilled beverage

Instructions:

1. The unsweetened almond milk should first be
    added to your blender.
2. The ripe banana should be peeled and added
    to the blender as well.
3. Greek yogurt (or dairy-free yogurt) should be
    added to the blender.
4. Rolled oats should be added because they are
    a great source of fiber and slow-releasing
    energy.
5. To add healthy fats and more protein, mix in
    some natural peanut (or almond) butter.
6. The chia seeds, which are rich in protein,
    fiber, and crucial omega-3 fatty acids, should
    be added.
7. It is optional to add honey or maple syrup if
    you like a sweeter drink.
8. Add the vanilla extract to the mixture for
    flavoring.
9. You can add a few ice cubes to the blender if
    you prefer chilly juice.
10. Then, mix everything until it has a smooth,
    creamy consistency.
11. Pour the protein power juice into a glass
    when it has been blended, then sip it.

This juice is an ideal post-workout beverage or a wholesome morning boost because it is loaded with protein, good fats, fiber, and critical elements. To add more nutrients and flavors, you may also add different fruits or vegetables like spinach, kale, or berries. Keep in mind that the sweetness can be changed to suit your taste. Enjoy your protein-boosting beverage!

Healthy Green Juice

Benefits

A type of green juice known as skinny green juice is mostly composed of green vegetables and is often low in calories. It is popular for its possible health advantages and is frequently included in healthy diets. The following are some advantages of drinking thin green juice:

Green vegetables are nutrient-dense and are abundant in important vitamins, minerals, and antioxidants. Examples include spinach, kale, cucumber, celery, and parsley. A concentrated amount of essential nutrients is present in skinny green juice, supporting general health and well-being.

Green veggies have a high water content, which aids in maintaining your hydration. For several body processes, such as digestion, skin health, and temperature control, adequate hydration is essential.

Weight management: As its name implies, slim green juice is low in calories and might be an excellent choice for people trying to lose weight or increase their intake of low-calorie foods.

Detoxification: By supporting the liver's natural detoxification processes, the antioxidants, and phytonutrients found in green vegetables can help the body detoxify.

An improved digestive system can be supported by the fiber content of green vegetables, which can facilitate digestion and encourage regular bowel movements.

Increased energy: Because slim green juice is nutrient-dense, it can provide you with a quick energy boost, making it a wonderful choice for an afternoon pick-me-up or a morning pick-me-up.

Enhanced immunity: Green vegetables include antioxidants that fight free radicals and support a robust immune system, lowering the risk of sickness.

Alkalizing properties: The alkalizing actions of many green vegetables on the body may assist maintain a healthy pH balance and lessen acidity.

Skin benefits: By preventing oxidative stress and encouraging collagen formation, antioxidants in green veggies can help you have better skin.

Even though slim green juice can be a healthy complement to a diet that is balanced, it should not take the place of entire fruits and vegetables in your daily diet, it is crucial to remember. For general health, it is crucial to eat a variety of fruits, vegetables, entire grains, and lean proteins. Before making big changes to your diet, it's also a good idea to speak with a healthcare provider or a qualified dietitian if you have any particular health conditions or concerns.

Recipe

Here is a straightforward and delectable recipe for a thin green juice:

Ingredients:

one cucumber
fresh spinach greens, 2 cups
1 apple green
Peeled half of a lemon
Fresh ginger, 1 inch long
(Adjust for desired consistency) 1 to 2 cups water or coconut water
Ice cubes, if desired

Instructions:

1. Thoroughly clean all the components.
2. Cut the cucumber into smaller pieces after peeling it.
3. Slice up the green apple after coring it.
4. Lemons should be peeled and then sliced into smaller pieces.

5. Ginger should be peeled and sliced into thin slices.
6. Combine the cucumber, spinach, green apple, lemon, and ginger in a juicer or blender.
7. Pour in the coconut water or water.
8. The mixture must be smooth. You can increase the amount of water or coconut water if you desire a thinner consistency.
9. If you want to make the juice cooler and fresher, you can optionally add a few ice cubes.
10. After blending, taste the juice and, if necessary, add additional lemon or ginger to customize the flavor.
11. For best freshness and nutrient preservation, pour the slim green juice into glasses and consume it right away.

Green juices should always be consumed fresh because oxidation causes their nutritious content to decrease over time. If you have any leftovers, you may keep them in the fridge for up to 24 hours in an airtight container. If there is any separation, give it a good shake before ingesting. Enjoy your slim green juice, which is both healthy and energizing!

Apple Pie Juice

Benefits

I may discuss the possible advantages of the main components of a classic pumpkin pie, which include pumpkin puree, spices (such as cinnamon, nutmeg, and ginger), and perhaps other ingredients like milk, eggs, and sugar. These advantages may not immediately apply to a blended juice product with those flavors as they are connected to the individual ingredients and are related with them:

Pureed pumpkin:
Beta-carotene, a precursor to vitamin A, which is necessary for healthy vision, the immune system, and skin, is abundant in pumpkin.

Fiber: Dietary fiber, which can help with digestion and increase a sensation of fullness, is present in pumpkin in good amounts.

Antioxidants: The antioxidants in pumpkin assist the body combat damaging free radicals, promoting general health.

Cinnamon:

Cinnamon has a lot of antioxidants that help shield the body from inflammation and oxidative damage.

Effects on inflammation: According to certain research, cinnamon may have anti-inflammatory characteristics that are helpful for a variety of medical ailments.

Nutmeg:
Support for digestion: Nutmeg has long been used to promote proper digestion and ease gastrointestinal discomfort.
Nutrients: The minerals manganese, copper, and magnesium are all present in nutmeg.

Ginger:
Ginger is renowned for its ability to reduce nausea and motion sickness.

Effects on inflammation: Ginger contains bioactive substances that have anti-inflammatory characteristics and may be helpful for some illnesses.

It's crucial to remember that although these ingredients may have health benefits, they are frequently utilized in pumpkin pies, which frequently include a lot of extra sugar and bad fats. In moderation, eating pumpkin pie can be delightful, but for optimum health, it is important to concentrate on eating complete fruits, vegetables, and a balanced diet.

It is crucial to review the components and nutritional details of any "Pumpkin Pie Juice" products you are thinking about purchasing to fully grasp the advantages and disadvantages. Making informed dietary decisions also means talking to a nutritionist or healthcare provider.

Recipe

A delicious way to savor the tastes of a traditional fall dish in liquid form is by making pumpkin pie juice. Here is a quick and tasty recipe for pumpkin pie juice:

Ingredients:

1 cup canned or homemade pumpkin puree

1 cup of apple cider or unsweetened apple juice
1/2 cup of your preferred milk, such as almond milk.
one ripe banana
1/8 teaspoon cinnamon powder
1/4 teaspoon of nutmeg, ground
1/8 teaspoon of ginger powder
1 tablespoon maple syrup or honey (modify to desired sweetness level)
Ice cubes, if desired
Whipping cream, as a garnish, is optional.
(Optional, garnish) Ground cinnamon or pumpkin pie spice

Instructions:

1. Blend the pumpkin puree, apple juice, almond milk, ripe banana, cinnamon, nutmeg, and ginger powders in a blender.
2. Blend the ingredients collectively and smoothly. You can add a bit extra apple juice or almond milk to the mixture if the consistency is too thick for your tastes.
3. Depending on your preferences, add honey or maple syrup to the juice to modify the sweetness. To integrate the additional sweetness, blend once more.

4. You can add some ice cubes to the blender and blend the juice until it is chilled if you like a chilled beverage.
5. Pour the pumpkin pie juice into glasses once you're happy with the flavor and consistency.
6. For an additional festive touch, you can add some ground cinnamon or pumpkin pie spice to the top of each glass before adding a dollop of whipped cream.
7. Enjoy the mouthwatering flavor of pumpkin pie in liquid form right away!

You are welcome to change the ingredients and amounts to suit your personal preferences. If you'd like, you can also add a tiny bit of vanilla extract for more taste complexity. The homemade pumpkin pie juice is delicious!

Mojito Juice With Mint

Benefits

I can tell you about the ingredients that are frequently found in a classic Mojito cocktail and their possible health advantages. Mint leaves, lime juice, sugar, rum, and soda water make up the traditional Mojito.

Menthol leaves

Digestive Health: Mint has a reputation for having carminative characteristics that can calm the digestive tract and ease indigestion or bloating. Mint may help to open up the airways and make breathing easier, making it beneficial for patients with respiratory conditions like asthma.

Antioxidants: Mint has antioxidants that can help the body fight off dangerous free radicals.

Citrus Juice: Lime juice is a great source of vitamin C, which is necessary for a strong immune system and healthy skin.
Lime juice includes antioxidants that, like those in mint, can shield the body from oxidative stress.

Sweetener (or sugar):
Energy: While sugar is a quick source of energy, it's important to use it sparingly to limit your intake of calories.

Rum (the alcoholic component of a typical Mojito):

Moderate Alcohol Consumption: Drinking alcohol in moderation may have some positive effects on the heart and social relaxation. However, drinking too much alcohol can have detrimental effects on your health.

Water Soda: Drinking soda water can help you stay hydrated, especially when combined with other juices and drinks.

While these ingredients may have some potential advantages, it's crucial to keep in mind that a Mojito drink frequently contains extra sugar and alcohol, which can negate the advantages and cause health problems if consumed in excess. A non-alcoholic version can be made with fresh mint leaves, lime juice, soda water, and a natural sweetener like honey or agave syrup if you're seeking a healthy alternative.

Recipe

A tasty and reviving beverage, mojito juice is ideal for hot summer days or any time you want a zesty treat. Here is a straightforward formula for minty mojito juice:

Ingredients:

1 cup of mint leaves, fresh
Fresh lime juice from one cup (approximately 6–8 limes)
1/2 cup sugar, taste-tested
2-cups of water
An ice cube
For decoration, use lime slices and mint sprigs.

Instructions:

1. The fresh mint leaves should be well-washed and dried.
2. The mint leaves, lime juice, sugar, and water should all be combined in a blender or food processor.
3. The mint leaves should be finely chopped and the mixture should be well-combined after blending the components.
4. When necessary, add extra sugar to the juice after tasting it to determine its sweetness. If

you want a tangier flavor, you may also add additional lime juice.

5. Use a fine mesh strainer to filter the liquid to get rid of any pulp or leftover mint leaves. If you want a drink that has more texture, you can skip this step.
6. Place ice cubes in serving glasses, then pour the mojito juice over the ice.
7. Add a lime slice and a mint sprig to the rim of each glass as a garnish.
8. Enjoy your revitalizing, minty mojito juice right away!

Note: To prepare a traditional mojito cocktail, add a little rum to each glass before serving an adult version. The non-alcoholic version is equally excellent, but this is optional.

You are free to modify the sweetness and lime intensity to suit your tastes. Take pleasure in your handmade minty mojito juice.

Coconut Cilantro Juice

Benefits

Combining cilantro (coriander leaves) with coconut juice or coconut water can result in cilantro coconut juice, which has several possible health advantages. It's important to remember that while cilantro is frequently used in cuisine and traditional medical procedures, there may not be much scientific research on the precise advantages of cilantro coconut juice. However, the following are some potential advantages linked to the specific ingredients:

Hydration: Due to its high water content and important minerals like potassium and sodium, coconut water is a naturally occurring electrolyte-rich beverage that aids in rehydrating the body. The maintenance of body processes and overall health depend on keeping appropriate hydration.

Coconut water is rich in nutrients including potassium, magnesium, calcium, and vitamin C, which are important for maintaining immunity, bone health, and a variety of biological processes.

Flavonoids and phenolic compounds, two types of antioxidants known to be present in cilantro, can aid the body fight off dangerous free radicals. This antioxidant function could improve general health and lessen oxidative stress.

Cilantro has historically been used for its potential detoxifying benefits. Although further research is required to prove cilantro's efficiency in this area, some studies have suggested that it may aid in the removal of heavy metals from the body.

Coconut water and cilantro both have the potential to improve digestive health. Fiber in coconut water helps maintain regular bowel movements, while cilantro has long been used to treat indigestion and enhance gut health.

Anti-Inflammatory: Linalool and eugenol, two ingredients in cilantro, have anti-inflammatory qualities. Although additional research is required to properly understand their effects, these qualities might help lower inflammatory responses in the body.

Cilantro has been shown in preliminary investigations to have antibacterial properties against specific bacteria and fungi. Coconut juice and cilantro may boost any potential antibacterial properties.

Although these advantages are linked to the individual components, the particular advantages of cilantro coconut juice as a blended beverage may differ based on the quantity of each component used and other unique aspects. As with any food or drink, moderation is necessary. Before introducing new foods or beverages to your diet, it's important to take into account any possible allergies or drug interactions. It's best to seek individualized counsel from a healthcare provider or a qualified dietician if you have any particular health issues.

Recipe

Here is a quick and tasty recipe for cilantro coconut juice that you can try:

Ingredients:

1 cup freshly cleaned and roughly cut cilantro (coriander) leaves

Coconut water, 1 cup

50 ml of coconut milk

1 tablespoon of either honey or agave syrup, taste-tested

Juiced lime, half

Ice cubes, if desired

Lime slices and fresh cilantro sprigs may be used as a garnish.

Instructions:

1. The cilantro leaves should be well-washed before chopping. For added flavor, you can utilize both the leaves and the delicate stems.
2. The chopped cilantro leaves, coconut milk, lime juice, honey, agave syrup, and coconut water should all be blended.
3. The cilantro leaves should be thoroughly incorporated into the mixture at this point.
4. If necessary, add extra honey or agave syrup after tasting the juice to get the appropriate level of sweetness.

5. If you would prefer a cold beverage, you can add a few ice cubes to the blender and pulse them into the juice until they are smashed.

6. If preferred, top up the glasses with a lime slice and a cilantro sprig after pouring the cilantro coconut juice into them.

7. Enjoy the zingy and tropical aromas of cilantro and coconut right now!

Note: You can strain the juice through a fine-mesh strainer before serving if you prefer a smoother texture. It's completely up to you; some people love the slightly pulpy feel of cilantro leaves.

You are welcome to change the components' amounts and ratios to suit your tastes. Enjoy your homemade coconut juice with cilantro!

Mix Of Fennel Juice

Benefits

The aromatic and tasty fennel plant (Foeniculum vulgare), which produces fennel juice, has several possible health advantages. Popular herb fennel is used in many dishes and traditional medical procedures. It concentrates many of its minerals and chemicals when juiced. While fennel juice may have some health advantages, it should be noted that it is not a replacement for medical care and that any serious health issues should be handled by a healthcare provider. Here are a few potential advantages of fennel juice:

Fennel juice has long been used to support digestion and treat related problems like bloating, gas, and indigestion. It could ease discomfort and relax the muscles in the digestive tract, making it easier for food to flow through.

Fennel includes several substances having anti-inflammatory effects, including flavonoids and polyphenols. Fennel juice regularly consumed may help lower inflammatory levels in the body, perhaps helping with ailments like arthritis and inflammatory bowel disease.

Fennel is a good source of antioxidants like vitamin C and flavonoids, which aid in scavenging the body's damaging free radicals. In addition to helping to reduce oxidative stress, antioxidants may also improve general health and well-being.

Fennel juice is thought to contain expectorant characteristics that can aid in removing mucus and alleviating respiratory disorders including coughs and bronchitis. This is thought to support respiratory health.

May Help with Weight Management: According to some supporters, the fiber component of fennel juice can aid in weight management by reducing hunger and fostering satiety.

Fennel includes phytoestrogens, which are plant chemicals with estrogen-like properties that may help maintain hormonal balance. Some people think fennel juice might balance hormones, especially in women who are going through menopause.

Oral Health: By preventing the formation of dangerous germs in the mouth, fennel's antibacterial qualities may help promote better oral health.

Fennel juice, like any vegetable-based juice, includes water and natural electrolytes, which can aid with hydration.

Despite these possible advantages, you should nevertheless proceed with caution, especially if you suffer from allergies or are taking any drugs. A certified dietician or a healthcare provider should be consulted if you're thinking about using fennel juice in your diet for certain health concerns to be sure it's safe and appropriate for you. Furthermore, moderation is essential because taking too much fennel or any supplement may have negative effects.

Recipe

Fennel juice is a tasty, refreshing beverage with certain health advantages. Fennel is popular for its licorice-like flavor and scent, which goes well with a variety of fruits and vegetables. Try this easy and delectable recipe for fennel juice:

Ingredients:

2 little or 1 large fennel bulbs
2 apples, green

one cucumber

1 lemon

Fresh ginger, cut into 1-inch pieces, optional (for extra zing).

Instructions:

1. Thoroughly clean all the components.
2. To fit in your juicer, slice the cucumber, green apples, and fennel bulbs into smaller pieces.
3. Remove any seeds by halving the lemon.
4. Peel and chop any ginger you use into smaller pieces.
5. Alternate the fennel, green apples, cucumber, lemon, and ginger (if used) as you feed the items into your juicer.
6. Give the juice a vigorous swirl once all the ingredients have been juiced to ensure that the flavors are evenly distributed.
7. Serve your juice over ice if you want it cooled. Otherwise, it's immediately ready for enjoyment!

The combination of fennel juice with other components, such as carrots, celery, spinach, or even a hint of mint, works particularly well. You are welcome to use your imagination and change the components to your liking.

Remember that the size and freshness of the vegetables you use can affect the juice's nutritional value and flavor. Before adding a lot of fennel or any new component to your diet, it's a good idea to speak with a healthcare provider if you have any particular health issues or diseases.

Liver Cleansing Tonic

Benefits

The detoxification processes and general health of the liver are supported by liver detox tonics, which are natural or herbal formulations. The liver is essential in the body's detoxification process because it processes and gets rid of medicines, poisons, and metabolic waste. Even while "liver detox tonics" have received little specialized scientific research, many of the individual substances that make up these tonics have been investigated for their possible health effects. The following are some potential advantages of liver detox tonics:

Supports Liver Function: Ingredients that support liver health and function are frequently found in liver detox tonics. These may include plants with hepatoprotective characteristics and the capacity to encourage liver regeneration, such as milk thistle (silymarin) and dandelion root.

Helps with Toxin Elimination: The liver is in charge of decomposing and getting rid of various toxins from the body. The liver's detoxification pathways are thought to be improved by ingredients like artichoke extract and turmeric, making it easier to get rid of dangerous toxins.

Reduces Oxidative Stress: Antioxidants like N-acetylcysteine (NAC) and alpha-lipoic acid, which can aid in reducing oxidative stress in the liver, may be present in liver detox tonics. The damage and impairment of liver cells are caused by oxidative stress.

Improves Digestion: Digestive herbs like ginger and peppermint are sometimes added to liver detox tonics to improve digestion and nutrient absorption.

Boosts Energy Levels: Liver detox tonics may improve general health and boost energy levels by aiding the liver's detoxification process.

Enhances Skin Health: Since the liver is involved in the body's toxin removal process, bettering liver function may also lead to healthier skin by reducing blemishes and acne.

Weight Loss: A healthy liver can help in metabolizing and processing fats more effectively, which may help with weight loss indirectly.

It's vital to remember that while liver detox tonics may have certain advantages, their efficacy, and safety will rely on the formulation and the user's specific health issues. To make sure a liver detox tonic is safe for you, it's a good idea to talk to a doctor before using it, especially if you have a history of liver disease, are pregnant or nursing, or take any drugs.

A balanced and healthy lifestyle is also necessary for promoting the health of the liver and general well-being. This includes eating a balanced diet, getting frequent exercise, and drinking alcohol in moderation.

Recipe

Please be aware that although the word "detoxing" the liver is frequently used in alternative medicine, it is crucial to keep in mind that the liver is already a very effective organ in the body's detoxification process. It's best to speak with a healthcare provider if you have any worries regarding the condition of your liver.

Despite this, some people include using homemade liver tonics in their daily health regimen. Here is a straightforward recipe for a liver detox tonic that uses all-natural components thought to boost liver function. It's critical to keep in mind that individual outcomes may differ and that this recipe shouldn't be used in place of seeking medical guidance.

Ingredients:

one medium lemon
one medium beetroot
Fresh ginger, 1 inch long
1 tablespoon of raw honey (to taste, optional)
water, 1 cup

Instructions:

1. To get rid of any residue or debris, properly wash the lemon, beetroot, and ginger.
2. Peel the ginger, and chop the lemon and beets into small pieces or slices.
3. Use a blender or food processor to combine all the ingredients, including the lemon, beets, ginger, and honey, if using.
4. Additionally, add the cup of water to the blender.
5. The combination should be blended until it forms a smooth, well-mixed liquid.
6. To attain the desired consistency, add extra water if the mixture is too thick.
7. Pour a glass or other container with the liver cleansing tonic.
8. It can be consumed right away or kept in the fridge for up to 24 hours.

9. It is advised to take this tonic empty-handed,
    preferably in the morning before breakfast.
    Vitamin C and antioxidants are provided by
    the lemon, and it is thought that the chemicals
    in ginger and beetroot may help to support
    the health of the liver.

Once more, it's important to approach "detox"
techniques cautiously and view them as a
component of a larger healthy lifestyle. Before
making any significant dietary or lifestyle changes,
it is essential to speak with a healthcare provider if
you have any pre-existing medical conditions or
questions regarding the condition of your liver.

Blast Of Beet Berry

Benefits

It sounds like "Beet Berry Blast" contains beets and
berries in some manner, probably as part of a
smoothie or drink. A delicious and healthy beverage
might be made by combining beets and berries, both
of which have several health advantages. The typical

components of a "Beet Berry Blast" may provide the following advantages:

Antioxidants: Fruits like blueberries, strawberries, and raspberries are abundant in flavonoids and anthocyanins, which act as antioxidants. These substances aid in the body's defense against dangerous free radicals, hence lowering oxidative stress and inflammation.

Nitrates, which are present in beets and which can enhance blood flow and lower blood pressure, are good for the heart. Beet nitrate consumption may promote cardiovascular health and lower the chance of developing heart disease.

Increases Immunity: Berries are renowned for having high levels of vitamin C, which is crucial for a strong immune system. Consuming meals high in vitamin C regularly can aid the body's defense mechanisms against infections and common diseases.

Supports Brain performance: Berries' polyphenols and antioxidants have been linked to enhanced memory and cognitive performance. They might lessen the chance of cognitive decline brought on by aging and assist in preventing damage to brain cells.

Berries and beets both have anti-inflammatory qualities that can help reduce the symptoms of inflammatory disorders and promote general joint and muscle function.

Beets include betalains, substances that aid in the body's detoxification process by supporting liver health and the removal of pollutants.

Berries are an excellent source of dietary fiber, which helps with digestion and fosters healthy gut flora. Additionally, high in fiber, beets support a healthy digestive system.

Nitric oxide, a naturally occurring substance found in beets, can increase blood flow and boost exercise performance. This might result in more energy and endurance for physical activity.

Skin Health: By lowering oxidative stress and shielding it from harm brought on by UV radiation and environmental toxins, the antioxidants in berries can promote healthier skin.

Beets and berries are both nutrient-rich foods because they both contain vital vitamins, minerals, and phytonutrients that promote general health and well-being.

Remember that the precise advantages of a "Beet Berry Blast" would depend on the particular components and their ratios. Although these foods have many health advantages, it is recommended to eat them as part of a balanced and diverse diet. If you have special dietary problems or medical issues, always seek the advice of a healthcare provider or nutritionist.

Recipe

Here is a recipe for a tasty Beet Berry Blast:

Ingredients:

1 medium-sized beetroot, cut after being peeled
1 cup of berries, all kinds including raspberries, blueberries, and strawberries
one little, ripe banana
1 cup of Greek yogurt, plain

(Or any other milk of your choosing) 1/2 cup of
unsweetened almond milk
Honey, 1 tablespoon (adjust to taste)
1 teaspoon of optionally nutritious chia seeds
Optional ice cubes for a cooler, thicker smoothie

Instructions:

1. Beetroot should be washed, peeled, and then cut into small pieces. You can pre-cook the beetroot until it's tender if you want a smoother texture.
2. Blend the banana, Greek yogurt, almond milk, honey, mixed berries, diced beetroot, and beets.
3. Chia seeds should also be added to the blender if you're using them.
4. Until the mixture has a smooth and creamy consistency, blend all the ingredients at high speed. You can add some ice cubes and combine the smoothie once more if you prefer it cooler.
5. Taste the smoothie and, if necessary, add more honey to change the sweetness.
6. The Beet Berry Blast should be poured into glasses and served right away. You may also

top it with chia seeds or some fresh berries as a garnish.

7. Take pleasure in your colorful and nourishing Beet Berry Blast smoothie! It's a delicious way to enjoy a refreshing treat while getting some beets and berries into your diet.

Juice of cucumber

Benefits

Due to its nutritious content and moisturizing qualities, cucumber juice provides several health benefits. Here are a few advantages of drinking cucumber juice:

Water makes up the majority of cucumber, making cucumber juice a refreshing and hydrating drink. The maintenance of physiological functioning and general health depends on staying hydrated.

Cucumber juice is nutrient-rich and contains important vitamins and minerals like potassium, magnesium, vitamin K, and vitamin C. These nutrients assist several body processes, such as muscle, immunological, and bone health.

Beta-carotene, flavonoids, and tannins, all powerful antioxidants, are abundant in cucumbers. By reducing oxidative stress and inflammation in the body and neutralizing dangerous free radicals, these antioxidants may minimize the chance of developing chronic diseases.

Skin health: The benefits of cucumber juice for the skin are well established. Due to its calming and cooling effects, it is frequently utilized in skincare regimens. Applying cucumber juice topically or utilizing skincare products containing cucumber extract may help lessen skin inflammation, puffiness, and redness.

Cucumber juice includes dietary fiber and water, which can help prevent constipation and encourage regular bowel movements, therefore it may help with digestion.

Weight loss: Because cucumber juice contains few calories, it can be a useful complement to a diet plan for losing weight. You can feel full and satisfied with fewer calories thanks to its high water content and fiber content.

Blood pressure control: Potassium, which is present in cucumbers, is essential for regulating blood pressure. Juice from cucumbers may enhance cardiovascular health when used in the diet.

Bone health: Vitamin K, which is crucial for bone health and may help to increase bone density and lower the incidence of fractures, is found in cucumber juice.

Cucumber juice can help to flush out toxins from the body and support kidney function because of its high water content.

Although cucumber juice has many health advantages, it should not be used as a substitute for a variety of full meals; rather, it should be included in a balanced diet.

Additionally, before making large dietary changes, anyone with certain medical issues or allergies should speak with their healthcare provider.

Consuming cucumber juice in excess might have some negative consequences, such as digestive distress or allergic reactions in sensitive people, therefore moderation is crucial.

Recipe

Here is a straightforward recipe for cool cucumber juice:

Ingredients:

(Peeled and chopped) 2 large cucumbers
Fresh mint leaves, half a cup
1 tablespoon sugar or honey, taste, and adjust
1 tablespoon of lemon or lime juice
125 ml of cold water
Ice cubes, if desired

Instructions:

1. Cucumbers should be well-washed, and peeling is optional. For simpler blending, cut the ingredients into smaller pieces.
2. The cut cucumbers and new mint leaves should be placed in a blender.

3. The cucumbers and mint should be pureed until smooth.

4. To separate the juice from the cucumber-mint puree, place a fine mesh strainer over a big basin or jug. To press down on the mixture and extract as much liquid as you can, use a spoon.

5. Save the remaining solids in the sieve and discard them or use them in other dishes.

6. To the cucumber-mint juice, add honey or sugar, and mix until it dissolves. Put as much sweetness in as you desire.

7. To give the juice a tart flavor, combine some lime or lemon juice.

8. Stir well as you add cold water to the mixture.

9. To chill the cucumber juice even further, if preferred, add ice cubes.

10. Add a slice of cucumber or a mint sprig as a garnish after pouring the cucumber juice into glasses.

11. Serve the cool cucumber juice right away and savor it!

12. You can change the sweetness, acidity, and mintiness to your liking. For further flavor variations, you can also add a dash of salt or

other herbs like basil. Enjoy the beneficial
effects of this tasty cucumber juice on your
health and hydration!

Thanks for reading. And more importantly, thanks
for getting this book.